UPDATED

Menopause, Naturally

PREPARING
FOR THE SECOND HALF OF LIFE

Sadja Greenwood, M.D.
Illustrations by Marcia Quackenbush

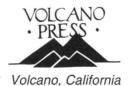

VOLCANO
· PRESS ·

Volcano, California

Library of Congress Cataloging in Publication Data

Greenwood, Sadja, 1930–
    Menopause, naturally : preparing for the second half of life /
Sadja Greenwood ; illustrations by Marcia Quackenbush. —
Updated and rev. 4th ed.
      p.   cm.
    Includes bibliographical references.
    ISBN 1-884244-05-X (trade paper)
    1. Menopause.   2. Middle aged women—Health and hygiene.
I. Title.
RG186.G74 1996
612.6'65—dc20   95-51147
                                                       CIP

Volcano Press participates in the Cataloging in Publication Program of the Library of Congress. However, in our opinion, the data provided us for this book by CIP does not adequately nor accurately reflect its scope and content. Therefore, we are offering our librarian/users the choice between LC's treatment and an Alternative CIP prepared by Sanford Berman, Head Cataloger at Hennepin County Library, Edina, Minnesota.

Alternative CIP

Greenwood, Sadja, 1930–
    Menopause, naturally. Updated: preparing for the second half of life.
Volcano Press, Volcano, CA, copyright 1984, 1989, 1992.
    PARTIAL CONTENTS: Sex in the second half of life. —Keep
your bones strong—how to avoid osteoporosis. —When periods
stop before 40. —Estrogen replacement therapy: the pros, cons,
and unknowns. —Beliefs about aging. —Relaxation: calming
down and letting go. —Use it or lose it: exercise in midlife.
    1. Menopause.   2. Middle-aged women—Health.
3. Osteoporosis—Prevention.   4. Middle-aged women—
Sexuality.   5. Holistic health.   6. Exercise for middle-aged
persons.   7. Estrogen replacement therapy.   8. Relaxation.
I. Title.
II. Volcano Press.   III. Title: Naturally, menopause.
                  618.175

Design/Production: David Charlsen
Composition: Jeff Brandenburg, ImageComp

Printed in the United States of America.

10 9 8 7 6

Volcano Press
P.O. Box 270
Volcano, CA 95689
Tel: (209) 296-3445
Fax: (209) 296-4515

CONTENTS

Author's Preface

My own menopause put me in awe of the human body. I marveled at the way the process of fertility, beginning around age 13, follows nature's plan and comes to a predictable close about 37 years later. I wanted to know more about these intricate mechanisms and lifetime purposes of our bodies, and how we could get in harmony with our changes.

These questions led me to set up a midlife and menopause service in a local women's clinic. I was struck by the complexity and diversity of each woman's menopausal experiences, and began to write guidelines for ways to stay healthy in midlife, emphasizing nutrition and enjoyable exercise. I realized that an individual approach to hormone use was also clearly necessary—but relatively complex. As I worked on these questions, the publisher and editor of Volcano Press suggested that I expand my guidelines into a book. This idea seemed absolutely right to me and the process began.

I am a general practice physician with a major interest in gynecology and women's health care, and an assistant clinical professor in the Department of Obstetrics, Gynecology, and Reproductive Sciences at the University of California Medical Center, San Francisco.

After practicing in a fairly traditional way for many years, and feeling perpetually stressed by the competing needs of work and raising children, I found a lump in my breast that turned out to be a cancer. I was in my early 40s at this time; the threat of death and the disfiguring treatment I underwent made me reassess my life in many ways. A patient for the first time, I understood the fear of disease, the power of modern medical treatment, and the awesome side effects they create. My reaction was to try my utmost to get healthy and stay that way. I have explored the values of nutrition, exercise, relaxation, meditation, imagery, and hope and humor, and have found that a great deal being written on these subjects is of relevance to the prevention and cure of disease. I have also discovered that many scientific reports on methods of self-care to promote health can be found in the medical literature, but are often ignored by doctors. We are so busy diagnosing and treating illness that we have no time to teach ourselves or our patients how to stay well.

As I approached menopause I realized that hormone use would not be in my best interest, as it might trigger a recurrence of breast cancer. For this reason I have had a special interest in safe, nonhormonal methods to lessen the symptoms of menopause and prevent the possible long-term results of a low estrogen level, such as fragile bones. Initially there were only anecdotal reports of such methods, but now many of these are documented in the scientific literature. I am not opposed to hormone therapy, and I have seen it bring relief and well-being to many of my patients. However, my major interest has been in health promotion, in the ways that we can help ourselves to feel well and remain vigorous with a minimum of medications. I have found that my patients and women attending my lectures are extremely interested in knowing more about effective methods of self-care. I see this book on menopause as an integration of my work with midlife women and my interests in the promotion of health.

So there you have it. I am a postmenopausal doctor, mother of two grown sons, a vegetarian, and a hiker, looking for the truths about life and the joy in every day.

In this updated edition of *Menopause, Naturally*, I have incorporated the changes in scientific knowledge since the revised edition of 1992. There is new material on the causes, prevention and treatment of osteoporosis, including nonhormonal methods of treatment. I have a new section on "phytochemicals," substances found in many vegetables, grains and fruits that give us some protection against heart disease, cancer, osteoporosis, and many other common diseases. The soybean turns out to be a powerhouse of phytochemicals for menopausal women, possibly helping with hot flashes, vaginal dryness and other problems. In many ways I consider this new information to be the most important in my book. I discuss natural progesterone—which is now available in pill form (although not yet licensed by the FDA). Women who experience unpleasant side effects with the synthetic progestins may feel better on natural progesterone. I have presented an up-to-date discussion of hormone replacement therapy, including an assessment of the many benefits and the risks of this therapy. Testosterone therapy is further discussed, as there is new evidence that use of this hormone may be harmful as well as helpful

The choice of whether or not to use postmenopausal hormones remains an important individual decision for each woman, based on her wishes, her age, her symptoms, her reactions to the medications, her family history, and her risk factors. The personal rating scale in Chapter 11 of this book is designed to help women make this decision. I see hormone replacement as valuable for some women and inadvisable for others. Doctors and nurse practitioners need to help each woman find the way that is the healthiest for her, without preconceived ideas that hormone therapy should be used by everyone, or that it is too dangerous to use at all. Natural alternatives to relieve symptoms and prevent the diseases of aging are emphasized throughout this book. My work is dedicated to helping women find their own way, so that they live the second half of life with knowledge and reassurance.

Many talks with midlife women, and my own experience, have helped me to see that while the hormone question is an important one, it is not the central issue for women as they age. Understanding oneself, building self-esteem despite becoming less sexually attractive, staying connected to the world, and nurturing one's creative outlets are the really important goals of midlife. I discuss these themes throughout the book. These aims are often accomplished by maintaining strong bonds with other women. I hope this book can act as such a bond with my readers.

I want to acknowledge the many people who have helped me with this book. First and foremost Ruth Gottstein, the publisher and editor of Volcano Press, and her colleague Leigh Davidson, have been incredibly supportive and helpful every step of the way. The wonderful drawings of Marcia Quackenbush inspire me to see the essence of people and the glow and humor in life. My companion, Alan Margolis, has given me unfailing encouragement and discerning suggestions from his extensive gynecologic background.

I want to thank the following physicians and scientists for their help, through their published work and via telephone calls: Winifred Cutler, Bruce Ettinger, Robert Heaney, Philip Hoffman, Morris Notelovitz, Diana Petitti, and Everett Smith. Thanks also to Dr. Ron Ruggiero for his great help in the area of pharmacology. Another thank-you goes to those who read and critiqued the book in its various stages—Joani Blank, Sally Campbell, Mary Davies, Neshama Franklin, Vicki Lansky, and Joan Robbins.

I also appreciate the medical library at the University of California Medical Center in San Francisco, and the people who work there, as extremely valuable scientific resources.

I also want to thank my mother for the inspiration of her example—she had more zest after menopause than most of us have in a lifetime; she showed me the positives and strengths of being a woman.

Finally, I must acknowledge the importance of my patients, especially those in the second half of life, for showing me the many facets of human experience and the need for an individualized approach to medical treatment.

Sadja Greenwood, M.D., M.P.H.
San Francisco, California
1995

PART I

The most creative force in the world is the menopausal woman with zest.

—Margaret Mead

Menopause: Fallacies, Facts, and New Possibilities *1*

*We are not troubled by things, but by the opinions which
we have of things.*

—Epictetus

*C*ecilia *walked rapidly into my office and pulled out her notes. "Look
at this record of my periods," she said with despair. "I'm probably
going through menopause at 42. It's ironic that I'll fall apart at a time
when I've finally found the right job and a good relationship." After
listening to Cecilia and examining her, I explained to her that her frequent
heavier periods were probably not a sign of impending menopause, but
might be related to a small fibroid tumor on her uterus, or to her increasing use of alcohol to calm herself after long hours of exacting work. I found
that she considered menopause to be a tragic time in life because of vivid
memories of her mother's problems after a hysterectomy at age 40. Her
mother's regrets over this surgical menopause had greatly influenced
Cecilia's early life.*

*Later in the same day Paula was telling me about her intense feelings of
irritability and depression before her periods. "Is this what it's like to go
through menopause?" she asked. "If so, I'm really dreading it."*

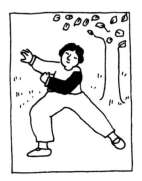

Neither of these women was actually going through menopause, but both showed me that they needed information and a more positive view about this natural transition between the years of fertility and the second half of life. Negative messages about menopause still abound in our culture—in cartoons and "old wives' tales"—despite all the recent attention to this subject. Fear and dread of the "change of life" are easy to acquire and can influence our behavior, our beliefs, and our bodies in subtly destructive ways.

Lillian, a Chinese-American woman of 50, viewed her menopause more positively. Her periods had stopped in her late 40s. Lillian said, "Getting rid of my periods was such a relief to me. I feel very balanced now. I took up Tai Chi about 10 years ago because I was getting sluggish, and that has made a big difference in my life. I do it every morning before work." Listening to Lillian made me reflect that she came from a culture with more respect for aging. She had also found a daily exercise that increased her strength and her feelings of inner harmony. Her menopause had been a smooth transition.

As a physician, I am always gathering information about the way people lead their daily lives and the way they feel about themselves. I have found that women who enter menopause viewing it as a natural process or transition have an easier time than those who view it as a crisis. If you exercise daily, eat healthy food, and work on achieving emotional balance you can usually manage to avoid many of the ills of midlife. One of

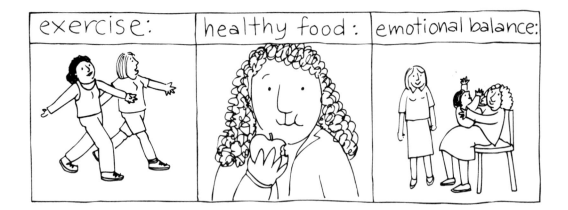

exercise: healthy food: emotional balance:

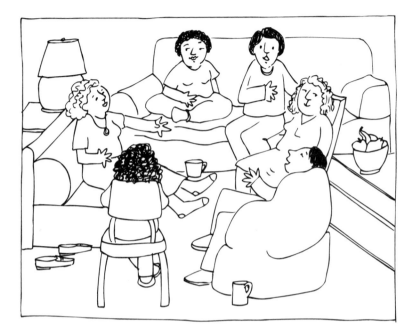

my patients recently told me that she "walked through menopause" by hiking every day in a state forest at a time when she
was out of work. Adopting such practices can cure many
problems more reliably than drugs or surgery. Skillful physicians can help their patients decide when self-care is sufficient,
or when medicine or live-saving technology is needed.

In recent years I have conducted special clinics for midlife
women and have taken part in numerous discussion groups
on menopause, sometimes including the women's husbands
or their male or female partners. I have always been impressed
by the help that people can give to each other in open discussions, and by the power of accurate, nonthreatening information.

What does happen in menopause? Strictly speaking, the
word "menopause" refers only to the final menstrual period.
In common usage, however, it designates a transitional time
from a few years before the last menses to a year or two after it.
As hormone output from the ovaries declines,
menstrual periods become irregular and then disappear.
Symptoms such as hot flashes, night sweats, and vaginal

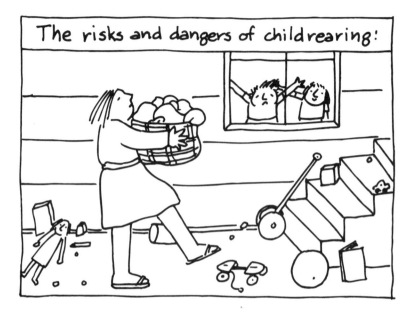

dryness are experienced at this time by four out of five women in our culture. (For reasons only partially understood, many fewer Japanese women experience hot flashes; as explained later in this book, the Japanese diet with its emphasis on soy foods may have something to do with this. Anthropologists report that rural Mayan women in southern Mexico do not even have a word for hot flashes, and speculate that this may have to do with frequent pregnancies and long periods of

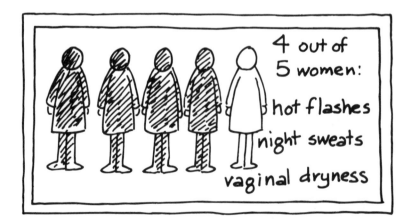

breast feeding.) Menopause usually occurs between ages 48 and 52, but it often happens earlier or later.

We don't know why menopause occurs in human beings but not in animals. Anthropologists have suggested that menopause has benefited our species during evolution, by releasing women from the stresses and dangers of childbearing to raise their late-born children and transmit cultural knowledge. They also point out that the menopausal transition is viewed very differently from one society to another. In western culture, with its strong emphasis on female youth and beauty, menopause is seen as a time of decline and loss of status for women. Belief in "progress" and in the taming and changing of natural forces makes us willing to alter women's hormonal levels in midlife. Menopause is viewed as a medical event—even a disease process—which requires treatment and careful medical followup. Other societies see menopause very differently. Among many nonwestern groups, older women enjoy increased status in the family and greater freedom in society at large. Menopause and the cessation of childbearing become positive events in their lives, and physical symptoms are given less attention.

Since the 1960s, profound changes have occurred in women's perceptions of their rights and roles in our society. Women are more active in every phase of community life, and more aware of their own needs and directions. This development has been linked to important changes in women's health care, including the ability to choose when or whether to have children, and a driving need on the part of many women to understand their bodies and participate in decisions about their own health or illness. Today, as the "baby-boom" generation begins to reach menopause, women are seeking new approaches to this transition. They want to replace negative stereotypes of menopause with a realistic and positive outlook, and they want to understand all possible options of traditional and alternative health care.

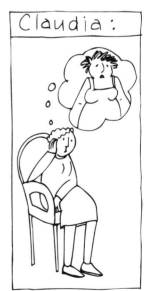

Claudia:

"You mean I don't have to go crazy in menopause?" Claudia laughed at herself as she asked this question, but there was an edge of fear in her voice. "Whenever I think of my mother and her depressions I get really

worried." When she analyzed it, Claudia wasn't so sure that her mother was more depressed in menopause than she had been years earlier or later. However, she had heard other relatives blame her mother's condition on "the change of life" and had accepted this explanation. Years later, as she approached menopause herself, she found that she had an irrational dread of reliving her mother's example. After a discussion and explanation of menopause, Claudia could see her own future as different from her mother's. She said that with her folk dancing and her counseling group, she felt she could get through just about anything.

Belle looked like she had a lot to say, and I listened intently to her story. "At first menopause was very difficult for me. I was waking at night with hot flashes and couldn't get back to sleep. I felt very self-conscious at work whenever I had one. My body seemed tired and tense, and I was getting depressed. My friend Janice had to drag me to her yoga class, but that was what really turned things around for me. I learned how to stretch and relax for the first time in my life. I started walking every day and eating a vegetarian diet. My hot flashes aren't nearly so bad when I exercise. I've learned so much in that class that I think I feel healthier than when I was 30." Belle did a yoga posture to show me how supple she had become. I was also impressed that her blood pressure was low and her heart rate slow and even.

I have two major aims in this book—to provide as much information as possible on how to promote good health and avoid illness in the second half of life, and to discuss some interesting and controversial questions about menopause such as how to deal with irregular bleeding, hot flashes and vaginal soreness, why mood swings may occur, how to make a personal and informed decision about hormone use, and how to avoid osteoporosis, heart disease, and other problems of aging with natural methods as well as with hormones.

Margaret Mead, the well-known anthropologist, spoke about postmenopausal zest, or PMZ. I've seen women who have PMZ and those who don't, and those who find it after a long process of self-exploration and self-healing. I would like to show you some signposts along the way.

The Hows and Whys of Menopausal Bleeding 2

"One month I can hardly get out of the house because of the bleeding I'm having, and the next month there's almost nothing. I never know what to expect these days."

"My periods are getting closer together and sometimes they are really heavy. Is that normal at 48?"

"Last month my period didn't come at all. I started waking up at night feeling really hot, and I couldn't get back to sleep. Then I had another period and everything is back to normal."

"My husband died when I was 49. It was a terrible time. I never had another period after his death, but I never had any menopausal symptoms either."

All these and many other patterns can occur in menopause. Let's review what is known about menstruation and its somewhat erratic behavior at this time of life. As the illustration on the next page shows, the uterus is a pear-shaped organ that develops a lining of cells and blood vessels every month in the fertile years. A menstrual period occurs when the uterus sheds this lining. This happens at regular intervals to most women under 45.

Each month the ovaries produce the hormones estrogen and progesterone in a predictable pattern. Estrogen is produced in the first half of the cycle in increasing amounts, causing a thick lining to grow in the uterus. At midcycle one

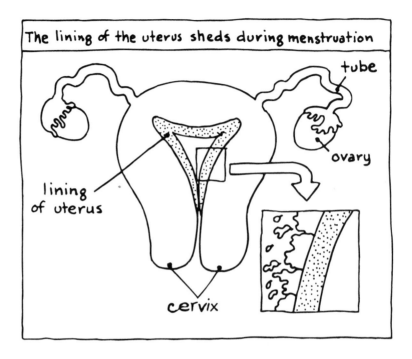

The lining of the uterus sheds during menstruation

tube

ovary

lining of uterus

cervix

ovary produces a mature egg cell, or ovum, which travels down a narrow tube into the uterus. This event is called *ovulation*, and marks the time when pregnancy can occur. After ovulation, in the two weeks before the next menstrual period, the ovary produces progesterone as well as estrogen. This causes the uterine lining to prepare for pregnancy by secreting special fluids and stabilizing the growth of the lining cells. When pregnancy does not occur, the ovaries stop their hormone production; estrogen and progesterone levels rapidly decrease, and the uterine lining loses its hormonal support and begins to break down. This lining is shed during the menstrual period, so the body can make a new nest for next month's egg cell. This is the monthly rhythm of women in their fertile years.

As women reach their mid-40s, on the average, ovulation becomes less regular, and hormonal output may vary. Many women notice that their periods are close together at this time, occurring every 21 to 25 days instead of every 28 days. The amount of bleeding may be lighter than before, but occasionally it is very heavy. Sometimes, when ovulation does not occur, a period is skipped. You may feel as if your period is coming for several weeks, with tender breasts or abdominal fullness, only to have these feelings fade away without a bleeding episode. Menses may resume in the next month or so.

Failure to ovulate can also cause prolonged "spotting" and erratic bleeding, since the ovaries do not secrete progesterone until ovulation occurs. In the absence of progesterone, estrogen levels tend to rise and fall and the lining is shed very irregularly. After a time of such erratic bleeding, ovulation may recur and normal periods are resumed.

Around the age of 50, menstrual periods will generally get further apart and become lighter, and then stop entirely. Some women experience this final pause before 50; some after. Very few women still menstruate at age 55. When a woman has had a year or two without bleeding at around age 50, she has completed the time known as menopause, and should sail smoothly into a new phase of middle life.

Many variations of bleeding patterns can occur as you enter menopause. Some are normal; others may indicate problems. It's typical for periods to be close together at first, with heavier bleeding from time to time. Timing may be unpredictable. Later on, periods become scantier in flow and further apart. Occasionally there is just spotting for a month or two. Some women abruptly cease menstruating, after a psychological shock or after stopping the birth control pill in their 40s.

The bleeding pattern most troublesome to women and worrisome to doctors is bleeding between periods, irregular periods that are close together, and very heavy bleeding. This can cause discomfort and anemia, and may be the result of hormonal imbalance, uterine fibroids, or cancer. Let us consider these factors and their treatment one by one.

HORMONAL IMBALANCE AND IRREGULAR OVULATION MAY CAUSE HEAVY BLEEDING

By far the most common cause of irregular bleeding among women in their late 40s is lack of ovulation and a resultant hormonal imbalance. When this situation occurs the cause is

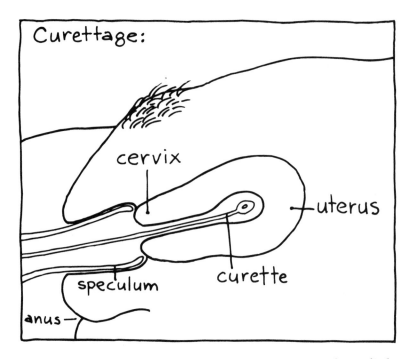

Curettage:

cervix

uterus

curette

speculum

anus

usually the production of too much estrogen and too little progesterone. There are various reasons for the problem, including the natural process of aging. However, frequently factors such as excessive stress can make the situation worse. Let's examine how this problem is usually treated, and then look at how it can be prevented from recurring.

When bleeding is prolonged or very heavy in the menopausal years, most doctors will first advise a minor operation to stop the bleeding and rule out cancer. Your doctor may advise an endometrial biopsy or a dilation and curettage (D&C)—in these procedures the lining of the uterus is removed, by suction or a scraping technique, and then analyzed for any abnormality. Some doctors also use a hysteroscope for diagnosis and treatment of abnormal bleeding; the hysteroscope is a long instrument with the diameter of a pencil, containing a system of lenses and a light source. It is inserted into the uterus through the cervix, enabling the operator to see the uterine lining and find the cause of the bleeding problem. These procedures can be done in a medical office or in an operating room where the patient can be put to sleep. If they are done in the doctor's office, the patient should take 400 mg of ibuprofen an hour in advance and have a paracervical block (local anesthesia of the cervix and uterus), because the procedures can be painful. Usually cancer is not found, and everyone is greatly relieved. However, after a D&C the uterine lining will grow back, and irregular bleeding may recur.

At this point the woman is often advised to take a hormone supplement called a *progestin*—similar to progesterone. Since progesterone, secreted by the ovary after ovulation, stabilizes the growth of the uterine lining, the use of a progestin usually stops irregular bleeding. The body responds as if ovulation had occurred. The progestin is taken for 1 or 2 weeks and when it is stopped, bleeding will recur, usually lasting less than a week, like a normal period. In many cases the irregular bleeding will not return in the next cycle. If it does, the progestin can be taken again. Occasionally the use of a progestin may cause feelings of fatigue, increased appetite, and other symptoms, but there seldomly are serious side effects.

Since many women would prefer to prevent such problems rather than take medicines when they occur, let's examine some natural remedies that make hormone imbalance and abnormal bleeding less likely.

Reduce emotional upsets

Emotional upset can have a profound effect on the reproductive system, causing little or no bleeding in some women and excessive or prolonged bleeding in others. Why is this so? In our long evolutionary history it has been better for the human species that fewer pregnancies occur in times of great social or personal disruption, or during prolonged episodes of exertion, exhaustion, famine, or fear. These protective mechanisms are still at work in our bodies. When we experience strong and prolonged negative emotions, the area in the brain that controls ovarian function may not operate well; ovulation may become irregular, and various hormonal problems can occur. Menstrual periods may stop completely or bleeding may be erratic and persistent. When the stressful situation is resolved, women often resume a more regular bleeding schedule. For older women, this will mean a smoother transition into menopause.

How do you resolve the stress of a serious family illness, an angry marriage, or overwhelming financial problems? Each of us must find our own way, giving ourselves time to consult our inner wisdom. Sometimes counseling is an answer; sometimes prayer or meditation; sometimes decisive action. When a start toward resolution is made, many disturbed body functions will improve.

Quit smoking

Smokers often have problems with abnormal bleeding. Substances in cigarette smoke, such as nicotine and carbon monoxide, enter the blood stream and are damaging to the ovaries, causing them to stop ovulating too early. Hence smokers enter menopause earlier than nonsmokers and may have a more difficult time. Cigarette smoking also affects the adrenal glands and the central nervous system, causing tension, rapid pulse, and easy exhaustion. All these factors make women more susceptible to irregular bleeding.

If you drink, be very moderate

Drinking alcohol in small amounts on social occasions is a pleasure for many people. However, alcohol in large quantities has a toxic effect on many body systems. It affects the ovaries, causing a decline in ovulation and hormone production. As a consequence, heavy drinkers often experience irregular and erratic bleeding, which usually clears up when the drinking stops.

As we age we are more affected by drugs of all kinds, including alcohol, because our bodies break them down and excrete them more slowly. In menopause it's wise to drink only small amounts (a little wine or beer on social occasions) and to quit entirely if you have bleeding problems.

Claire began to have extremely heavy and irregular periods at age 48. She worked as a waitress so she needed a lot of energy every day, but during her periods she felt exhausted. A discussion and physical exam revealed that she was very worried about money and was drinking too much. Her husband was out of work and they both drank beer all evening. They ate frozen dinners or cheese and crackers—whatever was easiest. Claire listened dubiously as I explained that alcohol, stress, and poor nutrition might be affecting her menstrual cycles. She tried taking progestins but the problem came back whenever she stopped. Finally her husband got a new job and decided to join AA. Claire went to some meetings with him and also decided to quit drinking. They both began to eat a healthier diet. In about three months Claire's periods were back to normal, and subsequently she started menopause without further problems.

Cut down on caffeine

We know a lot about the effects of caffeine (in coffee, tea, some cola drinks, and chocolate) on the nervous system, the heart, and the digestive system. It stimulates the brain to think more rapidly, banishes fatigue, and causes muscle tension. It stimulates the heart to beat more rapidly and forcefully, sometimes causing unpleasant feelings of pounding and skipped beats. It causes more acid secretion in the stomach, worsening the problem of ulcers.

But what does caffeine do to the woman's reproductive system? There is very little research in this area, but it is likely that excessive caffeine intake in midlife will cause constant feelings of tension and hypersensitivity to stimuli; this chronic stress can lead to disturbances in the output of hormones and to menstrual irregularities. Some women find that irregular heavy menstrual bleeding reverts to normal when they stop overstimulating their nervous systems with caffeine. Frequently people who drink a lot of coffee or tea also smoke cigarettes and then use alcohol to calm their "coffee nerves." The woman with bleeding problems needs to become free of dependence on all these drugs to establish a more normal menstrual rhythm or a smoother transition into menopause.

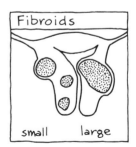
Fibroids — small, large

UTERINE FIBROIDS MAY CAUSE HEAVY BLEEDING

Some women in their fertile years develop irregular enlargements of the uterine muscle known as *fibroids* (also called myomas, or fibromyomas). Fibroids are almost never cancerous. Their growth is stimulated by ovarian hormones, especially estrogen. As a result, their growth generally diminishes in menopause as estrogen levels drop, and they actually shrink after menopause, rarely creating any further problems.

Some women who do not have distressing symptoms with fibroids are advised by their doctors to have the uterus removed simply because it is enlarged or "it is no longer a useful organ after childbearing is over." In such situations it is a good idea to seek a second opinion from another doctor, and to remember that the uterus will shrink significantly in size after menopause. Often it is possible to avoid surgery by simply waiting.

Some fibroids, however, enlarge to the size of a 5-month pregnancy or more, which can cause significant abdominal swelling and may place uncomfortable pressure on the bladder or bowel. Fibroids can also cause very heavy menstrual bleeding, which may result in severe anemia or make it difficult for a woman to carry on her daily activities. Profuse bleeding is often the result of so-called submucous fibroids, which lie just below the uterine lining and distort the normal shape of the uterine cavity. Any woman with very heavy periods should take supplemental iron, and have her doctor check her blood count at regular intervals. Sometimes medicines such as progestin, danazol, leuprolide (Lupron), or nafarelin (Synarel) are used to check heavy bleeding. Lupron and Synarel are powerful new medications that are almost identical to the brain chemical which regulates a woman's reproductive system. When used as a medicine they cause the ovaries to become quiescent and stop the secretion of estrogen. Heavy bleeding is checked, the uterus (with its fibroids) shrinks in size, and the woman may develop hot flashes and other symptoms of menopause. The ovaries resume their function when the drug is stopped. Generally, doctors use these drugs for only a few months to prepare a woman for surgery, to allow her to recover from anemia, and to make sure she bleeds less during the subsequent operation.

When bleeding or pain from fibroids is severe, many women opt for some kind of surgery. A variety of surgical treatments are currently available. If the woman wants to retain her uterus and her fertility, she can choose a myomectomy, a surgical operation in which the fibroids are removed but the uterus remains. This operation requires considerable technical skill on the part of the gynecologist, since it is important that all fibroids be removed, including very small ones that may be hard to detect. A picture of the uterus obtained by MRI (magnetic resonance imaging) is extremely useful to the surgeon, as it allows him or her to locate even very small fibroids. On rare occasions the operation becomes so technically difficult that the gynecologist is forced to do a hysterectomy after all, removing the entire uterus. After a myomectomy (or a hysterectomy) there is a 4- to 6-week recovery period before the woman has regained all her former strength. And there is a chance that the fibroids may grow back in future years, although this risk diminishes as the woman approaches her menopause. If menstrual bleeding was very heavy before a myomectomy, this situation is often improved after the operation. If the woman becomes pregnant, she may need to have a cesarean section for the delivery of the baby if the uterus has been significantly weakened by the myomectomy surgery. Myomectomy operations have become much more popular in recent years, as more women are waiting until 35 or 40 to have children, or are opting to retain their reproductive organs even if they don't want children.

Women with small fibroids and/or heavy menstrual bleeding have a simpler option: the permanent removal of the uterine lining and submucous fibroids (fibroids that bulge into the uterine cavity) through the hysteroscope. A hysteroscope is a pencil-thin operating tool that is inserted into the uterus through the vagina and cervix, so that no cutting is involved. The gynecologist is able to see the uterine lining and any submucous fibroids by means of a fiber-optic light source. The fibroids can be cut out with a wire loop and electric current.

The entire uterine lining can be permanently removed by means of an instrument called a *roller ball*. This is called "ablation" of the lining of the uterus (known as the endometrium). The woman is no longer fertile after ablation, and her menstrual periods thereafter will be very light or absent. The rest of the uterus remains intact, and the recovery period after this surgery is much quicker—the patient leaves the hospital within one day. Not all gynecologists have been trained in using these techniques; women who are interested should ask their doctor about this or call the nearest large medical center or medical school for a referral.

It is likely that fewer hysterectomies will be performed in the coming years as more doctors are trained to perform these operations which conserve the uterus. Women who feel strongly about conserving their uterus are generally pleased with these new procedures. However, other women may want or need a hysterectomy—because of cancer, severe pelvic pain or other serious conditions. If a hysterectomy is planned, it is important to discuss with your doctor the question of retaining your ovaries if the ovaries seem normal at the time of surgery. This allows for the continued production of ovarian hormones— estrogen, progesterone, and androgens in the premenopausal years—and thus enables a smoother transition into menopause when that time comes. Even after menopause the ovaries continue to secrete androgenic hormones; the importance of these hormones throughout life is discussed in the next chapter.

Another question to discuss with your doctor is banking your own blood in advance, so that it can be used if you need a transfusion. If you are not anemic you can bank several units of blood in the month before your operation, thereby insuring that you will not contact any virally transmitted diseases, such as hepatitis or AIDS, that are occasionally hard to detect in donated blood. The blood supply in the United States is currently well screened, so that the risk of contracting such diseases through a transfusion is very low. However, many people are deciding to bank their own blood in advance of elective surgery, to be absolutely safe. Be sure to take iron supplements if you are anemic—before and after banking your own blood.

The decision of whether or not to have a hysterectomy is a complex one, especially if the operation is not truly medically necessary. To clarify this point, a hysterectomy is often medically necessary for cancer, serious bleeding, overwhelming infection, severe pain, or other difficult problems. It is less necessary, or even optional, in many cases of fibroids or heavy bleeding that can be treated with progestins, other medications, or ablation of the uterine lining. If you are facing a hysterectomy you should fully discuss this with your doctor; all your questions should be answered. You should be aware that the uterus plays a role in some women's sexual response, discussed in Chapter 5 of this book. It may also protect premenopausal women against heart disease because of its production of a substance known as *prostacyclin*—which allows blood vessels to easily widen, and prevents too much blood clotting. In addition, there are emotional implications in surgery of any kind, some negative and some positive. Many women fear the idea of losing a part of their body, entering a hospital with its relative impersonality, and experiencing pain, weakness, and possible complications from surgery. Others welcome an immediate solution to their problems, and enjoy the special attention they receive in the hospital. Some people who dread an operation in advance feel greatly helped by it in the long run, while others feel angry or assaulted by their surgical experience. Much of this depends on the skill and caring of the doctors and nurses who attend you and the outcome of the surgery on health. As there are many unpredictables in this situation, it is best to have it well thought through in advance.

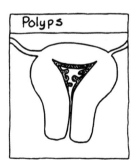

OVERGROWTH OR CANCER OF THE UTERINE LINING MAY CAUSE HEAVY BLEEDING

Unusually heavy, irregular, or persistent bleeding before menopause, or bleeding that occurs unexpectedly after periods have stopped for 6 months or more, may be due to overgrowth or cancer of the lining of the uterus. If blood loss is excessive or if cancer is suspected, doctors recommend a D&C to identify problems like polyps (usually benign, pod-shaped growths of the uterine lining) or hyperplasia (varying degrees of abnormality of the lining). Hyperplasia is not cancer, but a condition of overactivity of the lining cells. Occasionally cancer of the uterine lining is found, and surgical removal of the uterus (a hysterectomy) is recommended, along with other treatments.

However, much of the time the diagnosis is some stage of hyperplasia, which can usually be treated with a progestin, a medicine similar to progesterone. Progestin inhibits overgrowth of the uterine lining and restores a normal pattern to the cells when taken for 10 to 14 days each month or continuously for a few months. If your doctor has suggested a hysterectomy for a noncancerous condition such as hyperplasia, you can ask for a few courses of a progestin, followed by another D&C to assess the results. Sometimes the condition clears up very easily this way.

CANCER OF THE CERVIX MAY CAUSE HEAVY BLEEDING

Sometimes irregular bleeding is caused by cancer of the cervix—the lower part of the uterus at the top of the vagina (see picture on page 8). This problem is easily diagnosed by a Pap smear taken during a pelvic exam, which should be regularly continued during the menopausal years. Cervical cancer is preceded for several years by a condition known as dysplasia of the cervix, also identified by Pap smears. Dysplasia of the cervix is not cancer, but a precancerous condition of increased cellular activity, which sometimes becomes cancerous and sometimes returns to the original normal condition. Dysplasia almost never occurs in women who have never had intercourse, and is rare in women who always use a condom or diaphragm during sex, since the abnormality of dysplasia and cervical cancer is initiated by a factor that comes from a male sexual partner. This factor is suspected to be in certain strains of the sexually transmitted papilloma virus, which causes genital warts in men and women.

Women with dysplasia or cancer of the cervix should obtain prompt medical treatment, which may include further diagnostic tests, freezing or laser treatment of the cervix, removal of all genital warts, removal of a small part of the cervix by electrical excision or "cone biopsy," or a hysterectomy. If a hysterectomy is not required, shielding the cervix with a condom or diaphragm in every act of intercourse will minimize further exposure to the initiating factor. Male partners should be examined by a doctor for genital warts on the penis and inside the urethra, with the use of a magnifying lens and other diagnostic techniques. If the woman is a smoker, giving up smoking will also reduce the risk, since several studies have shown a relationship between cigarette smoking and cervical cancer.

There have been several studies showing that cervical cancer is less likely in women who take multivitamins and have a good intake of deeply colored and leafy vegetables. Folate (a B vitamin), beta carotene and vitamin C have been

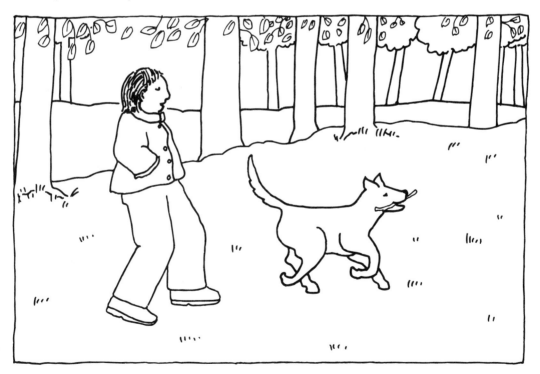

considered effective in prevention. Not all studies have confirmed this finding, but it is worth considering because you can rarely go wrong by eating more vegetables!

We have seen that bleeding problems in menopause are variable and affected by many factors. Some women have virtually no bleeding problems and others have erratic episodes of spotting or flooding or both. Since some bleeding difficulties are caused by serious problems such as uterine cancer, it is wise to regularly consult with your doctor. On the other hand, it is encouraging to remember that the vast majority of bleeding problems in menopause are the result of irregular ovulation and will be self-limited. The best method of prevention is paying attention to healthy living from day to day, as discussed in the second half of this book.

SOME POSITIVE ASPECTS OF MENOPAUSE, OR "THE END OF THE CURSE IS A BLESSING"

Menopause is not always a problem; let's remember the positive aspects of this transition. After menopause you have no more menstrual cramps, bleeding problems, or tampons and pads. You will have no more aching pelvic discomforts with and after ovulation, no more tender breasts before a period, and no more mood swings with premenstrual tension. You will no longer need to worry about endometriosis, fibroid tumors, birth-control devices, or unwanted pregnancy. Migraine headaches tend to disappear. Not all women experience all of these aggravations, but most of us have had some of them. Freedom from these difficulties is an aspect of menopause to be enjoyed.

> *"I tell you I will secretly dance*
> *and pour out a cup of wine on the earth*
> *when time stops that leak permanently;*
> *I will burn my last tampons as votive candles."*
>
> —*Marge Piercy**

From AVAILABLE LIGHT by Marge Piercy. Copyright © 1988 by Middle Marsh, Inc. Reprinted by permission of Alfred A. Knopf, Inc.

The Ovaries—Hidden Sources of Well-Being   3

J anet, a 45-year-old nurse, wanted a hysterectomy because of very large fibroid tumors that were causing pressure on her bladder. Her doctor said he would also remove both ovaries as a precautionary measure against ovarian cancer later on. "You're almost in menopause," he said, "so your ovaries won't be useful that much longer anyway." "Wait a minute," answered Janet. "I've always really liked what my ovaries have done for me. If they look normal, I want you to leave them in." Janet felt good about her decision, as she had read quite a lot about the low risk of cancer of the ovaries and the importance of these organs for general health and well-being. Her doctor found her ovaries were normal and did not remove them. Janet had a smooth recovery from her hysterectomy without needing to take any replacement hormones.

Throughout our lives our ovaries produce various hormones—estrogen, progesterone, and androgens—which influence general health, bone strength, sexuality, and reproduction. The

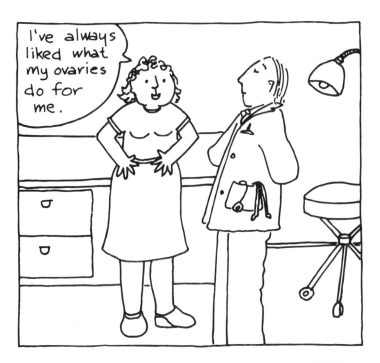

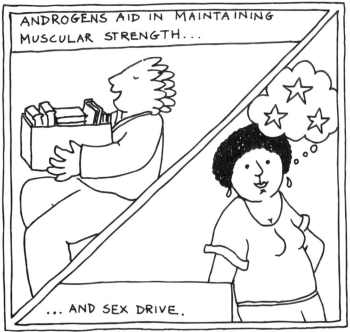

ovaries also produce a tiny egg cell each month during the menstrual years, which can develop into a baby when fertilized by a sperm.

As a woman approaches menopause these egg cells are produced less regularly. This causes changes in the timing and amount of her menstrual flow, as we discussed in the previous chapter. Finally, around age 50, no further egg cells are released. The woman's ability to bear children has ended.

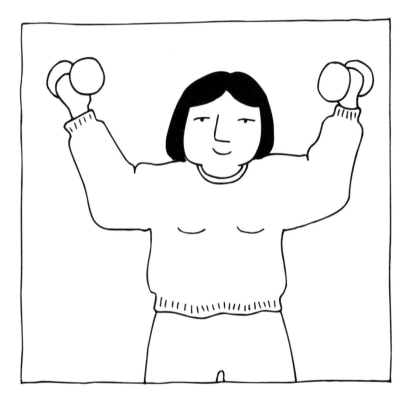

At menopause, when the ovaries are no longer producing egg cells, the secretion of estrogen and progesterone decreases greatly. However, the ovaries still play an important role at this time, because they continue to produce androgens, which influence general health and sexuality. Recent research indicates that androgens are secreted in small amounts even by women in their 80s. These hormones are similar to male hormones, but definitely belong in a woman's body. They aid in maintaining muscular strength, sex drive, and the elasticity of the vagina. Androgens are also secreted by the adrenal glands located above the kidneys. This adrenal output of androgens ensures that even women without ovaries produce some of these beneficial hormones.

Some androgens are converted to estrogen in the body's fat cells, so women with more fat on their bodies produce more estrogen after menopause, and may have fewer problems with hot flashes, vaginal dryness, and brittle bones. Here at last is an advantage to being plump!

But, as usual, the middle way is best. Being too fat has discomforts and hazards, including the risk of producing too much estrogen, which can cause cancer of the uterus (see Chapter 10). The best postmenopausal body is probably one that is shapely and very active. Women who are plump in the hips and thighs, but have a relatively smaller waistline, have less heart disease than women whose fat is in the upper abdomen. In other words, it is better to be a pear than an apple. A recent study of women, their weight, and their life span has shown that lean women, and those who have not gained more than 20 pounds since age 18, have the least chance of dying from heart attack, cancer and other diseases.

In the past many doctors felt they should routinely remove the ovaries of a woman over 40 if they had to remove her uterus. They reasoned that in menopause and beyond, the ovaries were useless organs which might become cancerous. The chance of a woman contracting cancer of the ovary in her lifetime is 1-2%. This risk is lower in women who have borne children or taken the oral contraceptive pill; it is also lower in women whose diet is low in animal fat and high in fiber. Risks are higher in families with frequent cases of ovarian cancer. Cancer of the ovary is hard to detect early and difficult to cure. Doctors reasoned that since they could give women estrogen pills to replace the hormones secreted by the ovaries, women would be better off without these organs.

New findings about postmenopausal ovaries are causing many doctors to change their views on the routine removal of healthy ovaries along with the uterus. The various hormones

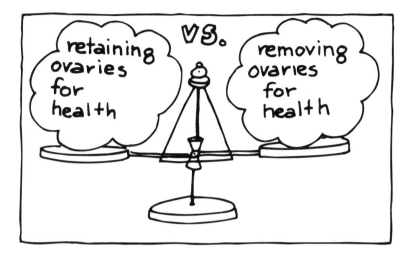

secreted by the ovaries in middle and old age contribute to well-being in many ways, and cannot always be duplicated by pills. For example, after ovarian removal some women find that estrogen pills do not restore their sex drive or their strength and well-being. What they are probably missing are the ovarian androgens, for these are the hormones most connected with sexual interest and response in both sexes. Testosterone, one of the main androgens secreted by the ovaries, has been used by women as a daily pill, a monthly injection, or an implant under the skin (renewed twice yearly). After ovarian removal, women who take androgenic hormones together with estrogen report increased sexual interest, energy and assertiveness compared to those taking only estrogen. However, there are drawbacks to testosterone replacement therapy, which are discussed in Chapter 10, including masculinizing side effects with large doses, an unfavorable effect on blood cholesterol and on the liver, and a possible increased risk of breast cancer. Some gynecologists prescribe 1% testosterone cream to be applied sparingly every other day to the clitoris and vaginal opening, which will usually increase sex drive without other side effects.

The argument for retaining the ovaries whenever possible should be balanced by the statement that in some cases the ovaries must be removed in surgery. For example, if they contain cancer, very large benign cysts, severe infection, or are a source of chronic pain, their removal may enhance a woman's health and chances for survival. Any patient facing a hysterectomy should carefully discuss this question with her doctor.

This discussion may not be easy. Many gynecologists still believe in the routine removal of ovaries after the age of 45 or 50, and some frighten their patients by saying they may get ovarian cancer if the ovaries are retained. However, recent studies indicate that the risk of ovarian cancer is actually lower than usual after a hysterectomy with retained ovaries. Women faced with this dilemma should carefully look at their own situation, and ask a lot of questions. Unless there is a family history of frequent ovarian cancer, the chance of getting this disease is about 1%. If the ovaries are not diseased they will continue secreting androgens for the rest of your life, which will help your bones, muscles, sex drive, and general well-being. If your gynecologist will not carefully listen to your concerns in this matter, you may need to seek a second or third opinion. While it is difficult to be at odds with your doctor, your wishes for your own body need to be respected.

While there are no foolproof methods as yet to detect ovarian cancer, radiologists have found that ultrasound is helpful. The ultrasound probe is often placed in the vagina to give the best results, especially if a large uterus blocks the ovaries from view by abdominal ultrasound. A blood test known as CA125 is also used to detect ovarian cancer, but it is not specific for this disease; fibroids, endometriosis and other conditions can interfere with the test.

MENOPAUSE WITH OVARIES BUT NO UTERUS

A woman who has had her uterus removed in her 30s or 40s, but still has her ovaries, may wonder how she will know when her "change of life" is occurring. When should she expect hot flashes? What if she never gets hot flashes? How will she know when to apply the principles discussed in this book, such as taking extra calcium, exercising, or considering hormone replacement?

Generally a woman with ovaries but no uterus goes through the menopausal transition like other women. She has no more periods but her ovaries continue to function like other women's until her late 40s. At that time, when she ceases to regularly ovulate and produces less estrogen, she may become aware of hot flashes, night sweats, and decreased vaginal secretions. If she has few symptoms of this kind (about 20% of women never get hot flashes), she can be fairly sure she has passed through the menopausal change somewhere between ages 48 and 53.

Some women who retain their ovaries after a hysterectomy do not continue to have normal ovarian function. They may experience vaginal dryness or hot flashes after the operation and enter menopause earlier than expected. The reasons for this are not entirely known—researchers have suggested that substances secreted by the uterus known as prostaglandins may play a role in maintaining ovulation. Also, surgery may partially interrupt the blood supply to the ovary.

Hormone therapy can be considered when symptoms occur or at age 50, whichever comes first. But no one should wait until a specific age to start exercising or eating foods high in calcium (see Chapter 7). Exercise is a good idea every day at every age. Calcium-rich foods are important for women throughout life, and calcium supplements can be started at 35 and then doubled at age 50 (see Chapter 16).

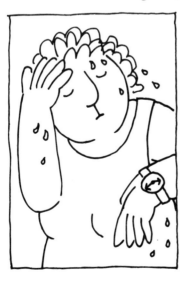

Hot Flashes — How to Live with Them or without Them

4

Hot flashes are the main signal of menopause in most western cultures, where a large majority of us experience them—sometimes mildly and sometimes fiercely. Women anthropologists have been studying menopause in many parts of the world, and report that in some cultures very few women are bothered by hot flashes. The difference may have to do with childbearing patterns and nutrition—scientists are currently thinking that the weak estrogen found in soybeans may protect Japanese and Chinese women from severe hot flashes. This theory is discussed later in this chapter and in Chapter 15. In our society, hot flashes can be very troublesome. We need to understand this phase of life, and learn how to get through it as easily as possible.

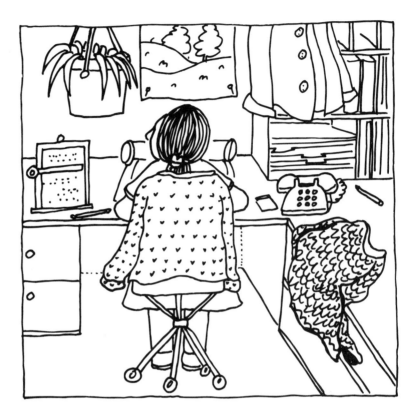

Women become more sensitive to temperature around the time of menopause. You may feel both cold and heat more acutely, and find you are frequently adding or removing sweaters. As menstrual periods cease, about 80% of us begin to experience hot flashes—feelings of extreme heat that come on unexpectedly. During a hot flash, the face, upper body, or entire body becomes very warm and flushed. Usually this feeling lasts for 1-5 minutes, but it can last longer. Sweating will also occur—sometimes a little and sometimes a lot. Before a flash begins, you can often feel it coming; you may need to take off your coat or sweater and fan yourself—which is understandable, since your skin temperature suddenly rises 7° or 8° F. However, the temperature inside your body does not rise, and no fever occurs. Your heart rate goes up during a hot flash, and you may feel breathless or dizzy. None of these symptoms are dangerous, but they can be very uncomfortable. Shortly after a hot flash the body temperature actually falls a little, and as sweat evaporates you may feel cold. Alternating between feelings of heat and cold is common in the menopausal years.

When hot flashes come at night, you may wake with feelings of breathlessness and heat. You may throw off your covers for a short time, and sweat a small or large amount. Waking with frequent flashes may interrupt your sleep, which can in turn produce fatigue and difficulty concentrating during the day. Some women are not aware of hot flashes at night but still report waking and not being able to go back to sleep. This menopausal insomnia can be a real problem, if you lie awake at two in the morning worrying about your life and its problems (which always seem bleakest in the early morning hours). Fortunately, these severe symptoms do not last long in most cases, and sounder sleep is usually restored after 6 to 12

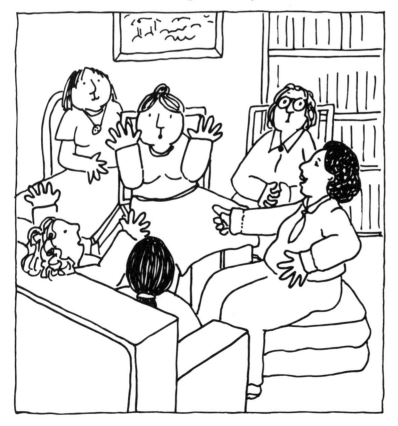

months. Sleep problems are usually less severe if you exercise during the day, take a warm bath or shower in the evening, avoid alcohol or caffeine with dinner, and have a glass of milk or some yogurt at bedtime. If you avoid milk products for any reason, try a little healthy carbohydrate-containing food, like a banana.

Hot flashes often begin when women are still having periods, typically during the days of menstrual flow. In general, they are most intense and frequent in the first two years of menopause, and then decrease in number and strength as the body gradually adapts to lower hormone levels and finds a new equilibrium. However, one-third of women still experience some feelings of heat as long as nine years after menopause.

Hot flashes need to be demystified. While they can be uncomfortable if a woman is overdressed and cannot shed some clothing, they need not be accompanied by feelings of embarrassment, anxiety, or helplessness. The popular image of the middle-aged woman as an emotional wreck, drenched in sweat and unable to cope, is part of the negative mythology of menopause. For the younger woman this inaccurate image creates fear and dread of hot flashes. For the menopausal woman the most distressing aspect of a hot flash often is her visibility during the episode—her fear that others are noticing her and making fun of or condemning her for growing older.

The group was talking about hot flashes. Marie said that her appearance was very important in her job as a designer, and her hot flashes had made her very self-conscious. She was greatly relieved when her doctor prescribed estrogen pills and the hot flashes went away. Sarah said that she had decided to live with the hot-flash situation and had brought a small fan to work so she could turn it on whenever necessary. Several younger women in her office had asked about it and appreciated her explanation of hot flashes. Susan said that she had three intense hot flashes during the group discussion and she wondered how bad she had looked. There was a brief silence; no one had even noticed.

Some women enjoy their hot flashes, feeling the heat as energy traveling through the body. Whenever I ask a large group of midlife women about their reactions to hot flashes, there are 2-3% in the audience who have a positive response! This potential for individual variability makes it important for each of you to be a student of your own responses, and not to automatically expect a negative experience.

WHAT CAUSES HOT FLASHES?

Hot flashes begin at a time in life when there is a relatively sudden decrease in estrogen output from the ovaries. The more gradual the decrease, the less severe the symptoms. If you have liberal amounts of body fat you may have fewer problems, as fat tissues manufacture more estrogen. On the other hand, if you are thin or have had your ovaries surgically

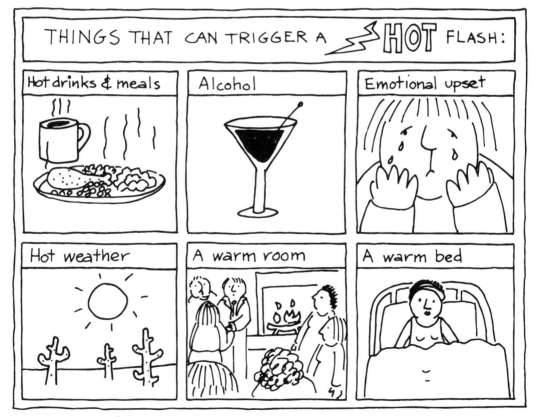

removed you may have more problems with hot flashes. Smokers often have more difficulty with hot flashes, because smoking reduces hormone output from the ovaries.

You can often come to recognize what brings on hot flashes, and this may be your key to controlling them. Emotional upset and stress, caffeine, hot drinks, hot meals, alcohol, hot weather, a warm room, or a warm bed all can be triggers. Studies on the timing of hot flashes show them to be most common in the late afternoon and early evening, with another peak in the middle of the night.

WHAT'S BEHIND HOT FLASHES?

The human body has several mechanisms to keep its internal temperature stable at an average 98.6° F. When the outside temperature is cold, we shiver and become pale. Shivering creates heat by contracting our muscles, and pale skin signifies that the body is keeping our blood warmer by contracting the skin's blood vessels and diverting blood flow to deeper tissues. When the outside temperature is warm, we sweat and flush, cooling ourselves as sweat evaporates and the skin's blood vessels expand, allowing more blood to lose heat to the outside. Before menopause these mechanisms are relatively subtle and continuous, so that women barely notice them unless the temperature is extremely cold or hot. Estrogen from the ovaries is believed to play a key role in helping the skin's blood vessels to expand and contract. Menopausal women, with less estrogen, cannot manage their temperature control as subtly. When a woman's body temperature goes up slightly, due to meals, hot drinks, or the normal afternoon rise in temperature, she intermittently cools herself by hot flashes and sweating. This theory seems to indicate that hot flashes are a necessary adaptive mechanism, with the purpose of maintaining the body's temperature within its normal limits.

Here is another interesting fact about hot flashes. Women who enter menopause in their teens or early 20s, because of genetic reasons or surgical removal of the ovaries, rarely have them. Hot flashes occur in these women only if they take supplementary estrogen for a time and then stop taking it. The trigger for hot flashes seems to be rapid withdrawal of estrogen from a body that has grown accustomed to it. After a number of years the body adapts and hot flashes become less frequent and intense.

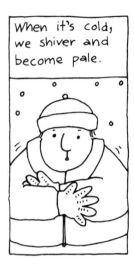

When it's cold, we shiver and become pale.

LIVING WITH HOT FLASHES

What does this tell us about living more easily with hot flashes? Since flashes accompany a rapid decrease in estrogen, avoiding lifestyle factors that contribute to this problem will help. Smoking and excess alcohol use interfere with ovarian function. Heavy use of marijuana and some other drugs may also affect hormonal output from the ovaries. Conversely, leading a healthy and drug-free life will permit the body to adjust more gradually to the menopausal process.

Exercise can be helpful in reducing the frequency and severity of hot flashes. Women who add brisk walking, jogging, dance or other sports to their daily routine may still have hot flashes but they are milder than those experienced by women who don't exercise. Several women have told me that they "walked through menopause"—walking every day for an hour or more, alone or with friends. This practice was effective in reducing hot flashes, elevating their mood and promoting sleep.

Regular self-calming is another helpful practice—through meditation, yoga, or silent prayer. A recent study from Wayne State University School of Medicine showed that women who were trained to do deep, slow abdominal breathing had a 40-50% decrease in hot flashes. They practiced slowing their breathing to 6-8 breaths per minute, and performed this technique twice a day for 15 minutes, as well as when they felt a hot flash coming on. Try breathing in for 5 seconds and then breathing out for 5 seconds and you will have the right timing. Put one hand on your abdomen and the other on your chest, and let the abdominal hand rise and fall with your breath,

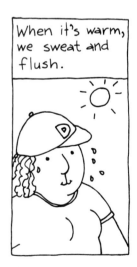

When it's warm, we sweat and flush.

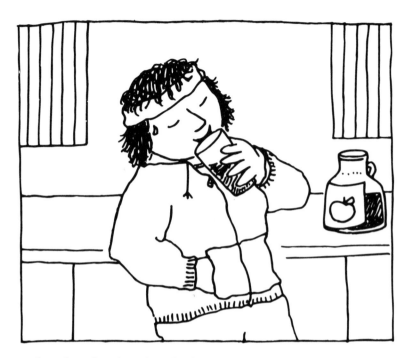

rather than the chest hand. This is what is meant by abdominal breathing.

In addition, menopausal women should not be underweight. As explained in Chapter 3, estrogen is actually manufactured in body fat from other hormones after menopause. A very thin woman will have less natural estrogen in her system, which may give her more problems with hot flashes.

Soybeans contain a substance that acts like a weak estrogen in the human body, so it is possible that drinking soy milk or regularly eating tofu will be helpful. Only about 10% of Japanese women who eat soy products such as tofu and miso on a daily basis are reported to have hot flashes, as compared to 80% of North Americans. See Chapter 15 for more information on soy foods and how to regularly include them in your meals.

Keeping cool is important for menopausal women, since all the precipitating factors in hot flashes are related to heat. Large meals, caffeine, alcohol, and strong emotions all make us warm. A menopausal woman reacts to heat by flushing and sweating in an exaggerated manner, so the most rational therapy for hot flashes is keeping cool. Carry a fan with you, the old-fashioned kind or a small, battery-operated one, and simply say "I'm having a hot flash" if you are asked to explain its use! Don't overdress, keep the house cool, eat frequent small meals, and go easy on caffeine and alcohol. Take a cool drink of water or juice after exercise. Sleep in a cool room. This will feel good and it really helps!

THERAPIES FOR HOT FLASHES

If a woman is severely troubled by hot flashes, she has several choices. She can wait for the flashes to decrease over time, which will happen naturally, or she can try estrogen therapy. The good news about estrogen supplements is that they are very effective in decreasing or eliminating hot flashes, night sweats and menopausal insomnia. Many women elect to use estrogen therapy for these reasons. However, these symptoms generally return whenever the drug is stopped. This return may be minimized if a woman tapers off her dose of estrogen very slowly, over a period of months. The decision of whether or not to take estrogen, with its various benefits and risks, is thoroughly discussed in Chapters 10 and 11 of this book.

Some doctors prescribe medicines other than estrogen for hot flashes. Natural progesterone pills can be taken, or a progestin such as Provera. This hormone also decreases hot flashes, but not quite as effectively as estrogen. Side effects like fatigue, weight gain, and depression can occur. Bellergal is sometimes suggested for women who cannot take estrogen—it is a combination of phenobarbital (a habit-forming sedative), ergotamine (which contracts smooth muscle and increases blood pressure), and belladonna (which inhibits the parasympathetic branch of the nervous system, causing dry mouth, dilated pupils, constipation, and rapid pulse). Bellergal has too many side effects for continuous use, but it is quite helpful at night if hot flashes cause severe insomnia. Clonidine (marketed as Catapres and Dixarit) is another treatment for hot flashes, although it is primarily used for high blood pressure. Clonidine

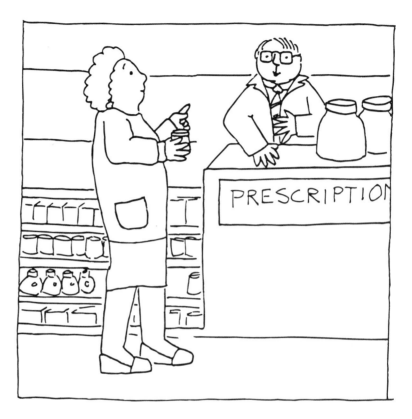

inhibits the release of norepinephrine in the brain. Side effects include sleepiness, dry mouth, and lowered blood pressure, but can be minimal in low doses. Clonidine is available as pills and in skin patches which will last up to a week. Low doses, .05 to .15 mg daily, are helpful to some women with severe hot flashes who should not or do not wish to take estrogen therapy. Clonidine is a prescription drug and should be used under the guidance of a physician familiar with its side effects.

It is important to remember that all medicines which are effective have many effects on the body besides the one intended. This is also true of recreational drugs, many foods and herbal remedies. Therefore, it is important to wisely use any medicine—only when needed, in the lowest effective dose, and for the shortest time that is necessary. Consult with your doctor or nurse practitioner to find out the reasons that any medicine is prescribed for you, and its potential side effects. Use your pharmacist as a source of information as well.

Some women are interested in alternative therapies for menopausal symptoms. Acupuncture, especially electro-stimulated acupuncture, has been shown to reduce the frequency of hot flashes. Many women have tried vitamin E in doses of 400 International Units (IU) once or twice daily and found this effective. Skin creams said to contain natural progesterone from plant sources are sold in natural food stores, and have become quite popular for the alleviation of hot flashes. They do seem to help some people; however, these creams are usually not adequately labeled, so the user does not know how much progesterone they contain, or how much she may be absorbing. They should never be used to balance estrogen if estrogen is also being used, as explained in Chapter 10. Homeopathic remedies, vitex agnus-castus and other American, European or Chinese herbal medicines may help. While there are numerous accounts of women who have been helped by these approaches, we do not yet have enough information on the doses and side effects involved. Like standard medicines, some may be helpful and others harmful. All such therapies should be approached with common sense and a positive but careful attitude. Listen to the wisdom of your body, and discontinue any therapy that causes unpleasant, unbalanced feelings.

Reliable and interesting information about botanical medicines can be obtained from publications of the American Botanical Council, P.O. Box 201660, Austin, TX 78720, telephone: 512-331-8868.

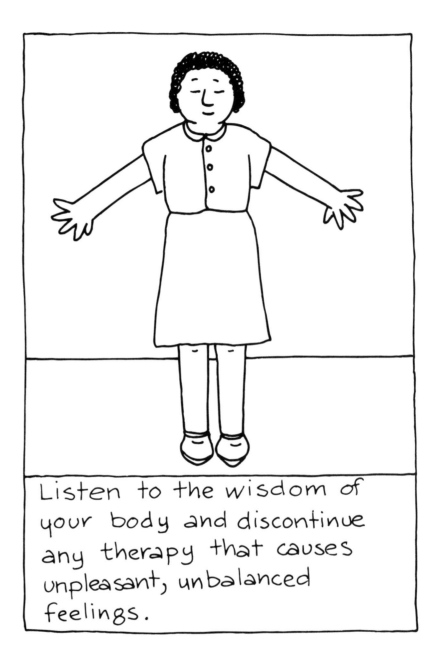

Listen to the wisdom of your body and discontinue any therapy that causes unpleasant, unbalanced feelings.

Sex in the Second Half of Life

5

The nutty thing about being an older woman as far as sex is concerned is that most women don't feel old when it comes to sex.

—*Rosetta Reitz*

Will menopause mean the end of your sexuality? Not at all. Menopause marks the end of your fertility, as your ovaries no longer produce eggs. However, you are still a sexual being, capable of giving and receiving love with body and spirit.

Sexual responsiveness changes with aging in both women and men. The sex drive may seem less urgent and arousal may take longer. However, many women continue to be sexually active into old age, both with partners and by masturbating. What is true in youth is equally true for older people—there is a tremendous individual variation in sexuality. Many women report being less interested in sex after the age of 50, feeling other aspects of their lives are more important. Others say sex is as enjoyable as ever. Some women lack a sexual partner at this time in their lives, when men their age may have sexual problems or are difficult to find. Some turn to other women for love and companionship; lesbian women report fewer problems finding a mate in midlife. Many older women masturbate for sexual pleasure.

Some women feel uneasy about masturbation, even in midlife. They were probably taught in childhood that it was dirty or sinful to touch their genitals, and the resultant feelings of discomfort lingered on. Perhaps this guilt can be lessened by the realization that most people masturbate, and the practice is helpful in maintaining sexual responsiveness in midlife. Masturbation has helped many people at times when they had no suitable sexual partners. It may even have saved a few people from unsuitable partners!

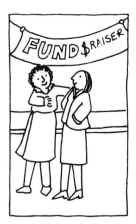

VAGINAL DRYNESS AND LOVEMAKING

"I finally met a really good man," said Diana. "We were both taking a class at the college extension. But when we got together to make love I felt extremely sore and I had to ask him to stop. He was worried that he had hurt me and I've got to do something to improve this situation. I really like him!" I examined Diana, who was 52, and found that her vaginal mucous membranes were thin and tender. I explained to her that she needed to use a small amount of estrogen cream on a regular basis, and a lubricant for intercourse. A few weeks later I bumped into Diana at a fund-raiser and she was radiant. "That situation is so much better," she said. "I feel really good about myself again."

The most frequent problem women in their 50s notice during intercourse is vaginal dryness and soreness. As estrogen levels drop during menopause and beyond, the vaginal walls become thinner and dryer. The cervix no longer secretes the quantities of mucous that it did during the fertile years. The entrance to the vagina becomes smaller, especially in a woman who has not borne children. As a result, intercourse can feel painful, even though a woman is sexually responsive and can easily achieve orgasm through stimulation of the clitoral area with the hand or mouth. Lesbian women usually have less difficulty with this problem because they may not use vaginal

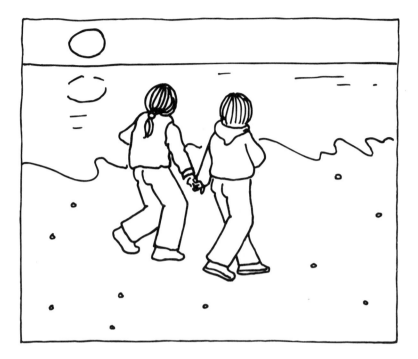

penetration in lovemaking, or may use a small object like a finger.

Several approaches are helpful. Couples should use lubricants during foreplay and wait until the woman is thoroughly aroused before vaginal penetration. Unscented creams or vegetable oils are useful, but should be avoided if the couple is using a condom to prevent sexually transmitted diseases, as they make condoms more likely to break. Water-soluble jellies or inserts are safe with condoms; these include jellies such as Lubifax, K-Y and Astroglide, and vaginal inserts such as Replens or Lubrin. These products are available in most pharmacies, or can be ordered through the *Good Vibrations Catalog* (see *Suggestions for Further Reading* at the end of this book). If the couple uses the woman-on-top position, she can control the rate of insertion of the man's penis and minimize any discomfort. Many women report that regular sexual activity, either masturbation or intercourse, helps reduce vaginal soreness. If these methods are not successful, a woman should talk to her doctor

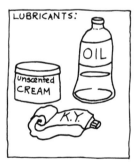

about using estrogen. She can take estrogen pills, wear the estrogen patch, or use a small amount of estrogen vaginal cream—as discussed in Chapter 10. This hormone will increase lubrication and thicken the vaginal lining, thereby reducing frictional discomfort or pain. A cream containing 1% or 2% testosterone can also help. Estrogen and testosterone creams are not designed as a lubricant for intercourse, and should not be used right before sex because they may affect your partner. If you are having any discomfort with intercourse, always use a lubricant at that time.

A recent study of women after menopause revealed that those who continued to have intercourse, or to masturbate, showed fewer signs of vaginal aging than sexually inactive women. The women who continued intercourse had similar estrogen levels but higher androgen levels than those who did not. The study appears to underline two important points. First, that continuing to be sexually active through intercourse or masturbation may help to preserve vaginal function after menopause. Second, that the ovaries—a major source of androgen secretion—remain active organs into old age.

What can couples do when their usual sexual activities become a problem? Frequently with aging the man may have

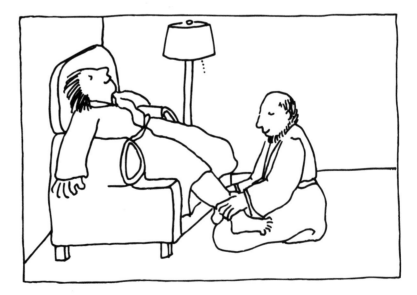

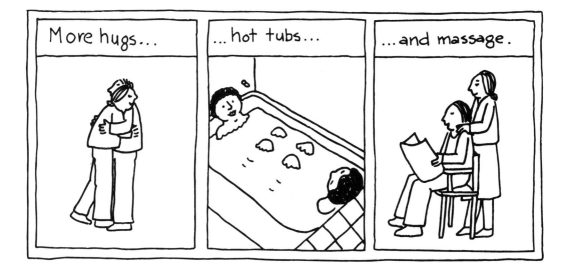

more difficulties with erection, or the woman with vaginal soreness. Illness or fatigue may impair the sexual response of one or both partners. Alcohol, tranquilizers and many medications can reduce sex drive and alter men's abilities to keep an erection. Such problems can be discussed with a doctor, as some people can decrease or eliminate medicines by making changes in eating and drinking habits, increasing exercise, and learning how to relax.

About half of women going through menopause notice a significant drop in their sex drive; reactions to this range from distress to acceptance to relief. Some women with decreased drive feel that they are entering a new phase of life, in which other interests and spiritual development can come to the forefront. It is important to acknowledge the choice not to be sexual as an important option for many women at different stages of their lives—an option which our culture does not value. On the other hand, some women find decreased drive to be a real problem, and for them the use of estrogen pills, the patch or vaginal cream is often helpful. Additionally, a small amount of 1% testosterone cream applied to the clitoris and surrounding area often increases sexual desire. This cream is used in small amounts, as described in Chapter 10; it must be

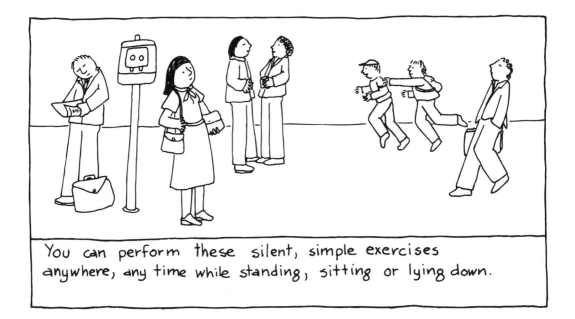

You can perform these silent, simple exercises anywhere, any time while standing, sitting or lying down.

prescribed by a physician and made up specially by a pharmacist in a vanishing cream base.

Midlife couples often come to realize that intercourse is not the only means of sexual expression. People give affection and pleasure to each other in many ways, and can stimulate one another with their hands, mouths, or a vibrator, and through massage with oils and creams. While the urgency to achieve orgasm may decline with age, the gratification of giving and receiving a loving touch remains strong. Learning how to give and receive a slow, deep massage of the hand, foot, shoulders, or entire body is a wonderful experience at any age.

One of the problems with sex in younger years for many women is the lack of prolonged caressing and foreplay, and the rapidity with which sexual encounters lead to intercourse. In later life there is an opportunity to correct this imbalance. Instead of giving up on sex, couples can include more touching in their lives, more hugs, hot tubs, and massage together, and expand their definition of sensual pleasure.

KEGEL'S EXERCISES

Squeezing and relaxing the muscles that surround the anus, vagina, and urethra (the opening for urine) can be very helpful. Women have found that these simple exercises increase their awareness of how to relax or to use these muscles during sex. Many have reported that it is easier to achieve orgasm after practicing Kegel's exercises. Other women say they have less tendency to develop hemorrhoids or to leak urine while coughing, laughing, or sneezing.

Kegel's exercises, named after the gynecologist who developed them to prevent urinary incontinence, are performed as follows: imagine that you want to stop urinating, and squeeze the muscles in your vaginal area firmly. Practice this squeeze technique while counting to 3—then relax for 3 counts. After repeating this squeeze-hold-relax technique a number of times, try a rapid alternation between tightening and letting go of the muscles. You can perform these silent, simple exercises anywhere and any time, while standing, sitting, or lying down. If you have trouble finding the right muscles to contract for Kegel's exercises you can use a device called Femina cones—a set of 5 tampon-shaped vaginal cones of increasing weights. You place the lightest one in the vagina, learn to contract your muscles to hold it in, and gradually progress to heavier cones.

INCONTINENCE, IRRITATION, AND INFECTION

Like the tissues lining the vagina, the lining of the urethra becomes thinner and less elastic after menopause. You may experience a need to urinate more frequently, or may have to go to the bathroom several times at night. Some women have difficulty with leakage of urine when they cough, sneeze, or laugh. Urinary incontinence should be discussed with a doctor, for there are several new approaches to treatment. Some medications predispose women to incontinence, especially a drug called Minipress given for high blood pressure. Kegel's exercises, and estrogen pills, patches or vaginal cream are often helpful. Bladder retraining is also useful—you learn to time your urination so that you go to the toilet every 2 hours during the day. In this way forgetful people will not have accidents because their bladder is too full, and women with an overactive bladder learn to increase the time between urinations. These methods are discussed in the very helpful book, *Staying Dry: A Practical Guide to Bladder Control*, by Kathryn Burgio and others. You can also get help by calling an organization known as *Help for Incontinent People* (1-800-BLADDER). As the vaginal tissues become thinner and dryer after menopause, they can easily be irritated by strong soaps. Warm (not hot) water is the best cleanser. For itching or irritated tissues, oatmeal baths are soothing (put some cooked oatmeal in a strainer and hold it under the tap as you fill the tub). Vaginal infections may occur after intercourse, especially with new partners, and often require a consultation with a doctor or nurse practitioner. Some women develop frequent bladder infections after menopause, due to changes in the kind of bacteria that live in the vagina and around the bladder opening. Small amounts of estrogen vaginal cream can restore the normal acidity of the vaginal tissues and help to prevent these infections. See Chapter 10 for a discussion of the various hormone creams your doctor can prescribe.

BIRTH CONTROL

How long should birth-control methods be used in the menopausal years? As long as menstrual periods occur and, to be on the safe side, for the next 6 to 12 months. However, the likelihood of becoming pregnant at around age 50 is small, so couples can use simple methods such as the diaphragm, condom, or foam. An IUD, if already in place and comfortable, may be left in until periods stop, but should be removed at that time or if heavy bleeding or pain occurs. Low-dose birth-control pills can be taken after age 40 if the woman is healthy and physically active. Smokers, however, should never take the pill after age 35, because of increased risk of complications such as heart attack or stroke. Women following fertility awareness methods of birth control may have difficulty recognizing ovulation, which occurs less regularly and with lessened secretion of cervical mucus.

Because of the risk of AIDS and other sexually transmitted diseases, everyone should be cautious with new sexual partners, or with an established partner who is not monogamous. You and your new partner should have an AIDS test before beginning to have sex together. Use condoms, or abstain from intercourse, until you are sure you both test negative for the AIDS virus and have committed to a monogamous relationship. Lesbian women have less risk in this regard, but should still discuss AIDS and be tested if necessary.

HYSTERECTOMY AND SEXUALITY

Women who are contemplating a hysterectomy for other than urgent reasons should get opinions from several doctors if possible, and should know that there are some sexual side effects from a hysterectomy.

While sexual pleasure leading to female orgasm is usually achieved from stimulation of the clitoris, the cervix and uterus also play a sexual role. To understand this sexual role of the uterus, we must reevaluate early theories about female response. Under the influence of Freudian theory, it was once believed that women who needed direct clitoral stimulation (as in masturbation or foreplay) to achieve orgasm were sexually immature. The "completely sexual" woman responded to intercourse alone, according to this view, which emphasized the importance of the "vaginal orgasm."

Many sexologists in recent years have pointed out that all female orgasms originate in the clitoris, which may be directly stimulated by hand or mouth, or indirectly by intercourse. Vaginal penetration is not necessary for orgasm, and by itself may not provide enough indirect clitoral stimulation for high levels of arousal. Psychologists and feminists have used these findings to counter early Freudian theories, and debunk the "myth of the vaginal orgasm." Now our views are changing again on this controversial subject! For many women there is something about vaginal penetration (along with clitoral stimulation) that enhances the quality of sexual pleasure and orgasm. Instead of intercourse, some women use fingers or other objects to achieve these sensations.

The extra pleasure may come not only from the physical closeness of vaginal penetration, but from the stimulation of the cervix and uterus. After a hysterectomy, this component is lost, as are the sensations from uterine contractions during orgasm. It is noteworthy that about one-third of women who have had a hysterectomy report that their sexual pleasure decreased after surgery.

Women considering a hysterectomy may be able to predict their own reactions in advance by self-observation. Women who find that cervical stimulation and/or deep thrusting greatly enhance the quality of their sexual pleasure may experience more loss after a hysterectomy. Conversely, those for whom deep penetration and movement in intercourse is painful may have better sex after a hysterectomy.

Until very recently, the uterus has been seen as primarily a reproductive organ without a sexual role. Now that we are more aware of its potential to enhance sexual experience, more research will appear to help women decide on the pros and cons of a hysterectomy.

European gynecologists have given more recognition to the sexual role played by the cervix, and will frequently perform a partial or subtotal hysterectomy when this operation is needed, removing the uterus but leaving the cervix and upper vagina intact. This operation has the added advantage of being simpler and quicker than a standard hysterectomy. However, the woman must continue to have regular Pap smears to detect cervical cancer.

If both ovaries are removed at the time of a hysterectomy, a woman's sexual response is often changed. Estrogen replacement will relieve hot flashes and prevent vaginal soreness, but it may not entirely restore the sex drive. Since estrogens differ somewhat in this regard, you should first try a few types of estrogen. Those containing estradiol may be the most helpful (see Chapter 10). It is not estrogen alone, but also androgenic hormones secreted by the ovaries and adrenal glands, which make a woman feel more sexual. Androgens such as testosterone can be given in pill form or by injection, and this treatment is often successful in restoring sex drive. However, the dosage used must be carefully monitored as increased facial hair growth or other masculinizing symptoms can occur. Recent research on possible problems with oral or injectable testosterone is discussed in Chapter 10. Small amounts of 1% or 2% testosterone vaginal cream have often been helpful as well. (See Chapter 10.)

These findings are causing many gynecologists to reconsider the preventive removal of healthy ovaries during a hysterectomy, even in menopausal women. For many years it was believed that any decrease in sex drive women felt after such surgery was psychological, and that all problems could be solved by counseling and estrogen. We are now less sure of these precepts and are coming to more fully appreciate the intricately connected wisdom of the body.

"I had to have it all taken out," explained Christie, "because I had a terrible infection in my uterus. But sex isn't quite the same as it used to be. I don't experience the same excitement at certain times of the month, and I miss the feeling of contractions deep inside. Still, I think I'm retraining myself to feel what I felt before." "How do you do that?" I asked. "I can't really explain it," she answered, "but I imagine what it used to feel like and try to match it." "Carry on," I said. We both laughed.

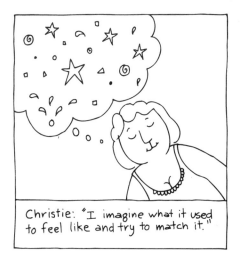

Christie: "I imagine what it used to feel like and try to match it."

Age Is Becoming . . . Your Looks in the Menopausal Years

6

After her husband died Eileen felt neutered inside. She found she had lost interest in her appearance and in trying to relate to men. She had felt gray inside and out for several years, until she met Jonathan in a folk dance class. He wasn't perfect; she would never marry him, but he helped her to feel alive again in an important way. She bought some new clothes and went to an exercise class. Her depression lifted and life began to glow. Her friends told her she looked wonderful. This is amazing, she said to herself. It's all still there, even at 55. This realization transformed her life in a subtle, positive way.

What will menopause do to our looks? Will the hormonal changes leave us fat, wrinkled, stiff, and sexually unappealing?

Not necessarily. Women who have an early menopause due to surgical removal of the ovaries at 25, for example, still look 25 despite their hormonal loss. It is not menopause but the aging process that most affects our appearance. Aging occurs at different rates in different people. Although genetic factors play a role in this, the crucial determinants of our appearance as we age seem to be health and happiness. We all get old and look old, but it can happen more or less beautifully, depending on our inner environment. Let's look at the questions about appearance.

WEIGHT GAIN

Weight gain often occurs at menopause but it is not necessarily inevitable. In our culture many people gain weight after the age of 30 because they slow down on exercise and eat too rich a diet. With aging we tend to reduce body movement more than food intake. At the time of menopause, the lowered output of sex hormones also affects body weight in several ways.

Studies done on menstruating women show they are more physically active in the first two weeks after their periods, when estrogen is the predominant hormone in their systems.

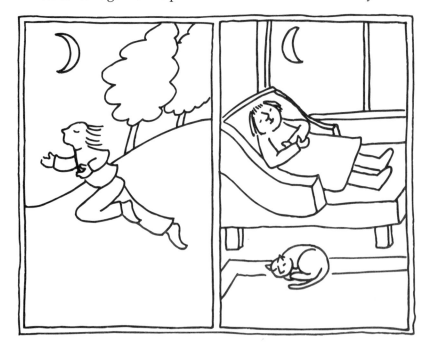

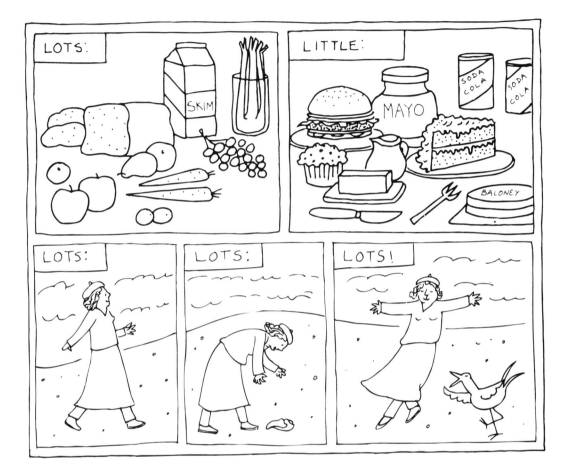

After ovulation, when progesterone is also produced by the ovaries, activity slows down and food intake increases; the body is preparing itself for pregnancy. Many women find they lose a little weight after menstruation and then gain weight before their periods due to these hormonal influences. For women on the birth-control pill, taking a progestin with estrogen for the whole month, weight gain is common.

But what about menopause? At this time estrogen levels fall sharply, and progesterone almost disappears from the system. We lose the subtle influence of estrogen to stimulate physical activity, and also the progesterone effect, which causes increased appetite and a slower pace. The net effect of the two hormones was to maintain weight levels, with a slight seesaw effect. After menopause, the seesaw effect is gone, and women approach a time of greater hormonal stability. However, recent studies show that they begin to lose their muscle mass at a faster rate, and gain fat tissue instead. As muscle mass goes down, there is a decline in the number of calories the body uses at rest—a fall in what is called the resting metabolic rate. Under these conditions weight gain is very likely unless you work to maintain muscle strength and change the way you eat. Maintaining your strength is discussed in Chapter 14—muscle-building, resistance exercises are the key. Changing the way you eat does not mean going hungry! It means eating lots of the right foods (whole grains, vegetables, and fruits) and as little as possible of the wrong foods (fats, sugars, refined flours, and rich meats). See Chapter 15 for nutritional advice.

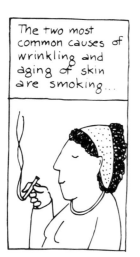

The two most common causes of wrinkling and aging of skin are smoking...

Women who take hormones during and after menopause often gain weight at the same rate as those who do not; the role of estrogen in this matter is not completely understood. The progestin that must be taken along with estrogen to prevent uterine cancer often causes a small increase in appetite and weight gain.

SKIN CHANGES

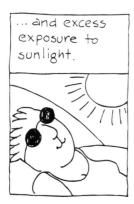

...and excess exposure to sunlight.

Another common concern about menopause is that the skin will become rapidly dry and wrinkled. In younger women the sex hormones produced by the ovaries have various effects on the skin. Estrogen has the effect of liquefying the waxy material produced in skin cells and thereby reducing the severity of blackheads and acne. Androgens, also produced by the ovaries, make acne worse. After menopause, when both hormones are reduced, facial pimples are rarely a severe problem. Estrogen also maintains the thickness of the skin in a woman's reproductive years, so your skin may gradually become thinner with aging. Menopause does play a part in this process, but the changes are gradual.

The two most common causes of wrinkling and aging of skin are smoking and excess exposure to sunlight. Smoking decreases blood supply to skin cells by constricting small blood vessels throughout the body. In addition, the blood of a smoker conveys less oxygen and more carbon monoxide than is normal. Skin cells and their underlying elastic layer are thus undernourished and lose their moisture and natural contour, resulting in wrinkles. After the age of 30 or 35, the skin of smokers and nonsmokers begins to look different. "Crow's feet" wrinkles around the eyes, lines and creases, and a blue-gray color due to poor oxygenation are all more apparent among smokers. The color difference can be reversed when smoking is stopped, but unfortunately the wrinkles remain.

Exposure to the sun is the most significant cause of skin wrinkling. People with dark skin are more protected from this effect and often have smooth, youthful skin into old age. Caucasians, with lighter skin coloring, are more prone to skin damage from sun exposure. Sunburn damages the elastic layers underneath skin cells, causing them to become less supportive of the skin itself. People who work outdoors all their lives often have more wrinkled, weather-beaten skin. They also are more likely to develop skin cancer. Some sunshine is healthy and promotes vitamin D formation in the skin, but sunburn can cause problems. Remember to wear a hat, protective clothing and sunscreen lotions outdoors.

Finally, general health and nutrition affect our skin as we age. Virtually all essential nutrients are needed for the health of our cover layer. People who ignore the precepts of healthy eating and living but take large amounts of one or two vitamins or minerals are not helping their skin and appearance as much as people who eat a variety of whole, natural foods and take a balanced vitamin/mineral supplement as needed.

Many people know vitamin A plays a role in the health of skin, eyes, and mucous membranes. However, this fat-soluble vitamin can be stored in the body, and excessive amounts from animal sources or vitamin pills can be dangerous. Most people should not take more than 15,000 IU daily as a supplement. The water-soluble form of vitamin A, known as beta carotene, is safe and useful. Best of all, get plenty of this nutrient from foods like carrots, sweet potatoes, yellow squash, yellow and red fruits, peppers, and all deep green, leafy vegetables.

Use of moisturizing skin cream is helpful for dry skin. Excessive hot water and soap wash away protective natural skin oils and should be avoided. Some cosmetics contain many chemicals which can be absorbed through the skin. Nothing will improve your appearance as much as a walk in the open air, healthy food, and activities that bring happiness and relaxation.

LOSS OF FLEXIBILITY

Changes in body flexibility—in the movement of joints and the elasticity of muscles—do occur with aging, but can be counteracted with stretching and exercise. It is not menopause that creates stiffness and joint pain so much as our habits of living, including insufficient movement, excess weight, and the wrong foods. A gradual program of stretching, such as yoga, and daily walking can restore a flexible body.

SEX APPEAL

Many women worry about losing their sex appeal after menopause. But sex appeal is a subtle force, made up of many variables, including interest in sexuality, transmitted verbally and by body language, and warmth and interest in others. These factors need not change with menopause. There are also hormonal factors which act as sex attractants in women. These sex attractants are known as pheromones; they exert their effects on men and women through subtle odors coming from the glands under our arms. The effects of pheromones can be easily seen in the animal world when a female is "in heat" and fertile, but in the human species today they operate mainly below our level of awareness. This source of sexual attraction is less potent after menopause; the effects of hormone therapy in this regard have not been studied. The pheromone responsible for sexual attraction has recently been synthesized in the laboratory by Dr. Winifred Cutler; it can be purchased, diluted in perfume and worn as a cosmetic by women to increase their sex appeal. We do not yet have any studies on its effectiveness, but interested readers can write to The Athena Institute, Dept. GLS, Haverford, PA 19041. The use of certain perfumes may stimulate the same areas in the brain as the pheromones do, giving out the same message of sexual receptivity. Among humans the most important sexual organ is the mind—most of

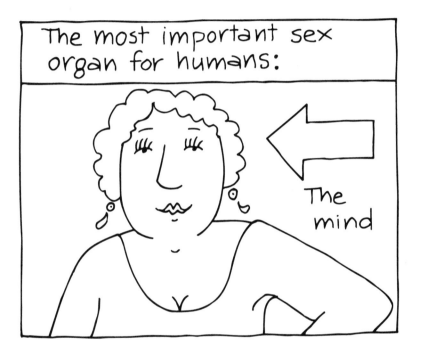

our turn-ons and turn-offs are related to our thought processes. If you are interested in sexuality, you can be sure menopause will not create a sudden end to your sex appeal.

The message of this chapter is that physical appearance does change with aging, but not markedly with menopause itself. The changes that come about with aging are minimized by healthy living and a sense of meaning in life, which is why some old people look young and—some young people look old.

Keep Your Bones Strong ...
How to Avoid Osteoporosis

7

After menopause women are more likely to develop osteoporosis—a condition in which bones lose their strength and fracture easily. "Osteon" is the Greek word for bone, and "porosis" means full of tiny holes, or porous. Bones which have osteoporosis are more likely to break, bend, or become compressed, leading to pain and disability.

THE BIOLOGY OF OSTEOPOROSIS

Why do older women develop osteoporosis? Throughout life our bones are constantly being remodeled—they are not inert organs despite their apparent rigidity. At certain times calcium is dissolved out of our bones to replenish the calcium supply in the blood, and in this process bone becomes weaker. This happens when our diets are too low in calcium and when we are physically inactive. Reducing diets are often deficient in calcium and are responsible for bone loss in many women. At other times increased amounts of calcium enter the bones from the blood stream, making them denser, stronger, and larger. This happens when we do physical work and exercise, and also when there is plenty of calcium in our diets.

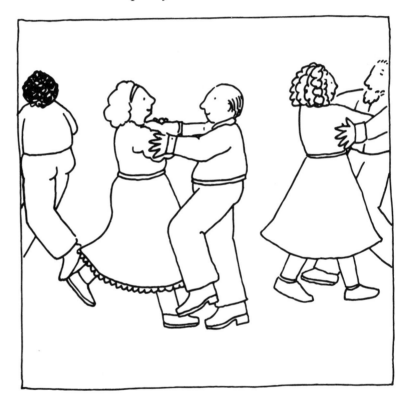

Erica was worried about developing brittle bones, or osteoporosis. Her mother had lost considerable height with aging and had back pain whenever she walked any distance. "What can I do if I don't want to take estrogen?" asked Erica. "I've heard that lots of calcium and a vegetarian diet are helpful." "You're right on that score," I said. "Another thing you can do is to exercise every day." "I haven't really exercised in years," groaned Erica. "Isn't it dangerous to start suddenly?" "Start with a walking program," I suggested, "and work up to 30 minutes a day at a brisk pace. Find something you really enjoy, like dancing or hiking, for the weekends. Start slowly and keep it up."

Calcium is a mineral with many functions. Besides giving strength to bones and teeth, it is dissolved in blood and body fluids where it plays a role in muscle contraction, the function of the heart, the transmission of nerve impulses, and the blood-clotting system. The body has many glandular systems which regulate and stabilize the calcium level in the blood, pulling it in and out of bones and in and out of our digestive tracts.

At the time of menopause there is a steep drop in estrogen production in women. Among its many functions, estrogen plays a major role in preserving bone strength. When estrogen is no longer abundant, bones dissolve more rapidly than they recalcify, and a woman's bones may become weaker and more likely to break. Why does estrogen play such an important role in keeping our bones strong? No one is sure, but it is probably a mechanism to protect the bones from excessive calcium loss during pregnancy, and to create rapid recalcification of bone between the end of breast-feeding and the next pregnancy. At these times estrogen levels in the body are high. While a woman is breast-feeding, her estrogen levels are low and calcium leaves the bones to go into milk formation.

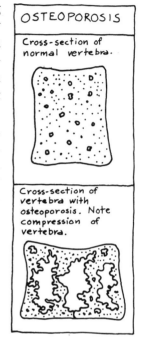

OSTEOPOROSIS

Cross-section of normal vertebra.

Cross-section of vertebra with osteoporosis. Note compression of vertebra.

After menopause, when estrogen levels drop, about 25% of White women develop serious osteoporosis. Asian women have a lower rate of osteoporosis than Whites, but are still at risk. Latina and Black women have the lowest risk; their darker skin color is believed to correlate with thicker and stronger bones. Susceptible women may fracture their wrists after a fall or milder trauma; this commonly occurs in the 50s. In their 60s, women may experience back pain as a result of the loss of calcium in their vertebral bones, with "crush fractures" or severe compression of these bones of the spine. Loss of height and a humped back may result. While about 30% of women show vertebral compression on X-ray films by age 70, severe pain or disability is rare; many women are not aware of having the condition. The most significant bone problem occurs typically after age 70 when fracture of the head of the thigh bone or femur, commonly known as fracture of the hip, may take place. Sixteen percent of White women will fracture their hip in their later years, and one-tenth of such patients will die from complications of the fracture. Those who recover are often permanently limited in their ability to walk without pain. Black and Latina women have a lower risk of hip fracture.

Osteoporosis can also cause tooth loss, which is more common in women than in men after age 50, and also more common in smokers. The weakened bone structure in the jaws of women with osteoporosis permits loosening and ultimate loss of teeth.

Clearly there are significant problems associated with osteoporosis in some older women. How can we identify those who are at risk of incurring fractures with aging due to osteoporosis?

WHO'S AT RISK?

A variety of X-ray techniques has been developed in recent years which are designed to screen women at the time of menopause, in order to identify those who are losing bone most rapidly and may therefore be most at risk for fractures. Tests called DEXA (dual energy X-ray absorptiometry) or DPA (dual photon absorptiometry) can measure the density of bone in the vertebrae of the low back and the hip. The other test is computed tomography or CT scan, which surveys the same areas using a different radiological technique. While both tests have certain advantages and disadvantages, I prefer the DEXA or DPA tests as they subject the patient to significantly less radiation than the CT scan. Ultrasound measurements of bone density may also become available in the coming years. A bone-screening test of your spine, hip, heel, or forearm will inform you and your doctor of your bone density compared to other women of your age and to women of 35—the age of maximum bone strength. Women with comparatively low bone density are more likely to suffer fractures later in life. If a woman has a bone-screening test at the onset of menopause and again a year later, the tests may help identify whether she is a rapid bone loser who could benefit from hormones, or a slow bone loser who might not need them to prevent subsequent fractures. However, not all women with low bone strength develop fractures. Hip fractures, for example, occur more often among older women who are prone to fall because of poor eyesight and the use of alcohol and tranquilizers. If your bone-density study shows low bone mass, you should take precautions against falls and trauma, as well as considering estrogen or other bone-building medications, calcium and muscle-building exercise.

Biochemical tests for prediction of rapid bone loss after menopause are also under evaluation, and promise to be less expensive than X-ray studies. Measurements of calcium and other products of bone breakdown in the urine can be helpful in determining who is at risk. At present most of these tests are only beginning to be used, so their validity in predicting fracture rates is still under investigation.

We should also look at genetic and lifestyle factors—such as race, body build, and use of alcohol or cigarettes—to help decide who is most at risk for brittle bones. The table on page 66 summarizes these factors, which will be discussed individually. Read the table with care, noting how it applies to you.

Genetic and medical factors
White women are at the highest risk for osteoporosis, followed by Asians. Latina women from Central America have a lower risk of fracture. Black women develop the problem less often, perhaps because of heavier bones or favorable hormonal differences. However, a recent study done in New York and Philadelphia showed that Black women who are thin, who drink more than 7 drinks a week, or have had a previous stroke are at increased risk for hip fracture.

Women who have had a previous fracture that occurred easily—from a minor fall, light blow, or twisting motion—may already have some osteoporosis.

Women with female relatives who had hip fractures or significant height loss with aging may inherit a family tendency toward osteoporosis. A genetic marker for osteoporosis, related to the vitamin D receptor in cells, has recently been found.

Women who are slim, with small muscle mass, are more at risk of osteoporosis than heavier, more muscular women. This is especially true if they are short and thin, as their total body weight is less. Several reasons are obvious here—more weight means more gravitational pull on the body and more work for the bones and muscles—all of which keep the bones calcified. More fat means more estrogen production within the body which helps prevent osteoporosis (see Chapter 3). The slender smoker is at greatest risk, and the obese nonsmoker at lowest risk of bone fractures.

Women with an earlier menopause often have more osteoporosis, since they lose bone over a longer period of time.

Patients with chronic diarrhea, such as ulcerative colitis or Crohn's disease, absorb less calcium and lose more in their stools. The same problems can occur if part of the intestinal tract has been removed by surgery. Patients on kidney dialysis can develop calcium deficiency and need special care for this problem. Patients who use cortisone daily in significant amounts develop osteoporosis. Women on daily doses of thyroid higher than needed for replacement, or on Dilantin or aluminum-containing antacids, are also at risk.

Factors That Increase Your Risk of Osteoporosis and Fractures

Genetic or Medical Factors

Light-colored skin

Previous fractures that occurred easily, without major trauma

Female relatives with osteoporosis

Being thin (especially if you are short)

Early menopause

Chronic diarrhea or surgical removal of part of the stomach or small intestine

Kidney disease with dialysis

Daily use of cortisone

Use of thyroid hormone in high doses, Dilantin, or aluminum-containing antacids

Lifestyle Factors

High alcohol use

Smoking

Lack of exercise

Low-calcium diet

Lack of vitamin D from sun, diet, or pills

Very high-protein diet

High-salt diet

Never having borne children

High caffeine use

Lifestyle factors

Let's look at lifestyle—the daily habits that cause osteoporosis, as well as those that increase bone strength.

High alcohol use contributes to osteoporosis and bone fractures. Excess alcohol is toxic to the ovaries, causing infrequent ovulation and menstrual irregularities in younger women, as well as decreased breast size. The menopausal woman who heavily uses alcohol may have less hormonal output from her ovaries, and as a result can have more problems with hot flashes and rapid loss of calcium from her bones. Many people who heavily drink do not pay attention to their diets, which compounds the problem of loss of calcium from bones. Finally, heavy use of alcohol leads to accidents, falls, and fractures. Many hip fractures in older women are caused

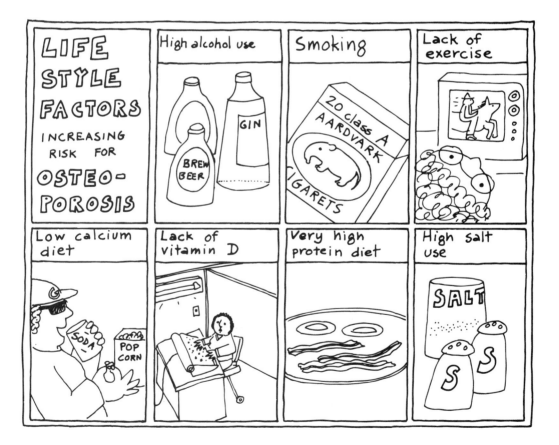

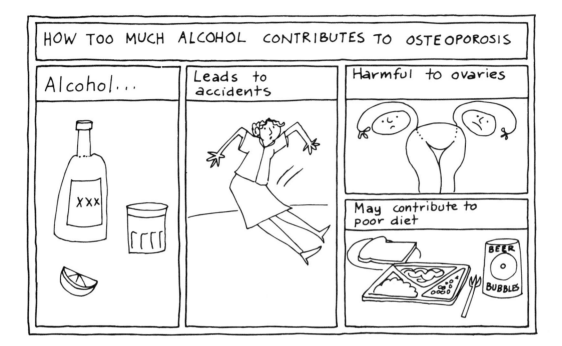

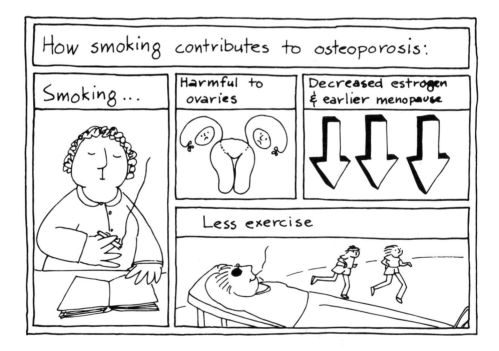

by falls related to the use of alcohol or tranquilizers. Although heavy drinking is clearly injurious, recent studies show moderate social drinking may be favorable for bone strength! Women consuming 1 or 2 drinks a day seem to have better bone density than abstainers; this may be because alcohol increases the conversion of adrenal androgens to estrogen in body fat (see Chapter 3).

Smoking contributes directly to osteoporosis. First of all, smokers have a decreased estrogen level in their blood and an earlier menopause. Smokers reach menopause with bones that are already weaker than nonsmokers. Several studies have shown higher rates of bone fractures in postmenopausal smokers, probably because of harmful effects of smoking on the ovaries and the parathyroid glands in the neck which regulate calcium levels in the blood. Since smokers tend to weigh less and exercise less than nonsmokers, their risk of osteoporosis is also higher on this account. Thin smokers are at special risk for fractures.

Lack of exercise can cause osteoporosis. When people are inactive during illness, their bones will lose calcium just as their muscles will become weaker. Conversely, when we walk, run, jump, dance, or otherwise jar our skeletons, a mild electrical energy charge develops along the bone which stimulates bone growth and calcification. Bones get stronger and thicker when the muscles attached to them are vigorously exercised. When exercise stops, muscle and bone strength will be lost. That is why you should exercise at least 3 times a week. Our arms as well as our legs need exercise to keep our bones strong. Tennis players have significantly thicker bones in the arm that holds the racket. Similar effects can be achieved through energetic gardening, lifting, working out with weights, and other upper-body exercise. Jogging or walking while moving the hands holding small weights is also useful; this form of exercise is called "heavy hands."

A recent study done at Tufts University looked at postmenopausal women who regularly walked a mile or more a day, either at work or as recreation. These women were found to lose bone more slowly than sedentary women, both in the hip and all over the body. Because of this, they had up to 7

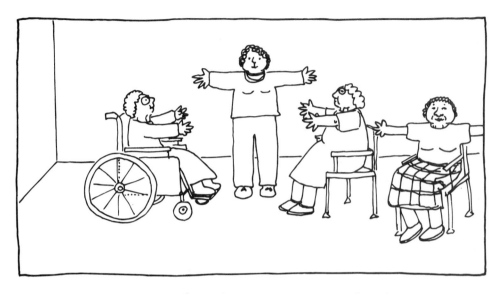

years more bone in reserve, meaning that they would take substantially longer to reach the time of bone fragility when fractures can occur. Most people can walk a mile in 20 to 25 minutes; brisk walkers do it in 15 minutes, and race walkers in 10 to 12. Another study from Tufts showed that postmenopausal women who did muscle-strengthening exercises twice a week for 40 minutes were able to gain a small amount of bone in their hips and spine over the course of a year. They improved their strength and their balance as well. The moral of this story is clear—find a way to walk every day, and work out with weights, such as 5- to 10-pound dumbbells, at least twice a week.

A very interesting study was done at the University of Wisconsin by Dr. Everett Smith. He studied women in a nursing home, average age 80, by measuring the size and calcification of their bones with an X-ray technique. One group of women exercised their arms and legs for 30 minutes, 3 times a week sitting in their chairs; a second group took extra calcium; and a control group made no changes in their diet or exercise. While the control group lost bone calcium during the three years of the study, the exercise group and the calcium group both gained bone, the exercise group most of all. When you consider that these women were about 80 years old and exercised from their chairs, the results are very encouraging. Exercise programs for the elderly can help to gain independence, restore the ability to walk, and prevent falls and fractures. But don't wait until you are elderly to begin; start today!

Clearly, part of the current problem of osteoporosis is related to our sedentary lives and our reliance on motors instead of feet. Women who leave all the "heavy work" for men are not using their bodies enough or doing the best for their bones. Exercise should be a lifelong commitment, planned for every day. Chapter 14 gives more suggestions on how to begin and maintain a joyous and self-perpetuating plan for movement.

A low-calcium diet can also contribute to osteoporosis. Young women who eat fast foods, sodas and chips fail to get enough calcium—since our peak bone mass is achieved at age 30, it is especially important to get adequate calcium early in life. Elderly people who subsist on tea, toast, lunch meat, and canned fruit are also in short supply of calcium. Since many other nutrients found in plant foods also help in bone strength, our diets should always be rich in vegetables, fruits and whole grains. Magnesium is an important element for bones, and is found in all plant foods, especially beans. New research indicates that weakly estrogenic substances in the soybean may be especially helpful (see Chapter 15).

Calcium is contained in many common foods which should be consumed regularly by women of all ages. If you eat plenty of foods containing calcium in your teens, 20s, and 30s, and exercise regularly, you will reach menopause with bones of maximum strength. But even if you haven't paid much attention to calcium in your diet up to now, begin at once! As the table on the next page shows, a wide variety of foods are good calcium sources; you can get plenty of calcium from healthful and tasty foods even if you don't like milk products. Calcium-fortified orange juice is now on the market, providing as much calcium per ounce as milk. Studies indicate that this calcium is well absorbed.

Many other foods are also good sources of calcium. However, spinach, chard, beet greens, parsley, rhubarb, and

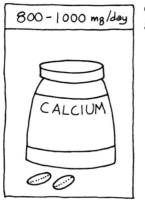

chocolate are not included here since their calcium is poorly absorbed due to their oxalic acid content.

Common Foods High in Calcium

Food	Amount	Calcium Content
skim-milk powder	¼ cup	400 mg
1% fat milk	1 cup	350 mg
calcium-fortified soy milk	1 cup	300 mg
yogurt	1 cup	300 mg
low-fat cottage cheese	1 cup	120 mg
collard greens, cooked	1 cup	360 mg
sardines, canned	8 medium	350 mg
blackstrap molasses	2 tablespoons	280 mg
sesame seed meal (tahini)	¼ cup	270 mg
kale, cooked	1 cup	200 mg
salmon, canned with bones	3 ounces	170 mg
broccoli, cooked	1 stalk	160 mg
tofu (soybean curd)	4 ounces	150 mg
corn tortillas	2	120 mg
calcium-fortified orange juice	1 cup	320 mg

When making soup stock from bones, add 1 or 2 tablespoons of vinegar during the boiling process. The acid in the vinegar will dissolve the calcium out of the bones, providing a soup stock unusually rich in calcium.

Doctors at the National Institutes of Health believe that young women, ages 11-24 should get 1,200 mg of calcium per day, women ages 25-50 should get 1,000 mg, and women over 50 should have 1,500 mg daily. Since most people get 400-500 mg per day from food, calcium supplements are often necessary. They generally come as 250- or 500-mg tablets, and are best absorbed if taken with food. Calcium in the form of calcium carbonate or calcium citrate is easily found in pharmacies and health food stores. Calcium citrate dissolves very quickly in the stomach, and calcium carbonate comes in a chewable form which is dissolved in your mouth. You can test one of your regular calcium carbonate tablets by dropping it into a glass of plain vinegar; it should have dissolved within 30 to 40 minutes. If it has not, switch brands—you may not be absorbing your tablet. See Chapter 16 for further details about calcium supplements.

Whether a high-calcium diet at the time of menopause will protect against bone loss has been debated by many researchers. Ideally, the high-calcium intake should have started many years earlier, to enable women to reach menopause with maximum bone strength. When estrogen levels drop off at menopause, bone loss is accelerated in most women. Calcium and vitamin D supplements started at this time are not as effective as estrogen in preventing bone loss, but they do have some protective effect and should be used by most women.

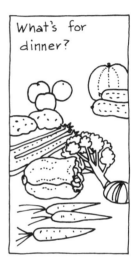

Vitamin D must be present in the body to allow absorption of calcium from the intestine. This vitamin is formed on bare skin when we are outdoors in the sun. It is stored in the liver until needed, and then changed in the kidneys to its active form. However, many people are cut off from the sun by clothing, remaining indoors, long and dark winters, window glass, or smog. Others rightly fear that excess sun exposure may cause skin cancer or more rapid aging of skin. For these reasons vitamin D has been added to many milk products; 8 ounces of fortified skim, low-fat, or whole milk provides 100 IU of vitamin D. Older women should get about 400 IU of vitamin D daily to ensure optimum calcium absorption. This is most easily done by taking a daily multivitamin supplement containing vitamin D. Large doses of vitamin D, over 800 IU daily, can be toxic to the liver and should be avoided. Several recent studies have shown that vitamin D, taken along with calcium supplements, reduces the risk of fractures in older women.

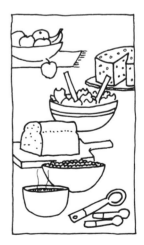

A very high-protein diet is one which contains twice the body's daily need for protein—eggs for breakfast and meat, fish, poultry, or dairy products at other meals. Eating like this is common in western countries; many people consider such food indispensable for health, and a symbol of good living. Some dieters subsist mainly on protein-rich foods. While small amounts of protein are essential, large amounts can cause problems. Animal foods are often high in fat and can lead to obesity and heart disease. In addition, they play a role in the osteoporosis story. The end products of digesting protein-rich foods are acids, such as sulfuric acid, which the body excretes in the urine. In response, the kidneys excrete calcium to balance this acid. Even young people eating a very high-protein diet lose significant amounts of calcium in their urine. The postmenopausal woman is most at risk from this dietary cause of calcium loss, because of her lack of estrogen with its protective effect on bones.

Bone studies on elderly women eating high-meat diets (the Eskimo), mixed diets (the average American), and vegetarian diets (Seventh-Day Adventists), show that high-meat eaters have the most osteoporosis, and vegetarians the least. Nutritional research indicates that the postmenopausal woman should not emphasize flesh foods, but concentrate on eating whole grains, vegetables, fruits, and beans (with an emphasis on soy products—see Chapter 15). In middle age and beyond, women and men can lower their risk of osteoporosis, heart disease and cancer if they try new answers to the question, "What's for dinner?"

A diet high in salt (sodium chloride) is detrimental in several ways. It has long been known that too much salt can lead to high blood pressure in susceptible people. Recently it has also been found that salt has the effect of causing the kidneys to excrete more calcium in the urine. Over the long run such urinary loss of calcium can contribute to osteoporosis. Dramatic decreases in urinary calcium have been documented in patients with kidney stones when they reduce their salt intake.

Women who have never had children have more risk of osteoporosis, because the high hormone output in pregnancy contributes to bone strength. While this is true in western countries, where pregnancies are limited in number and dietary calcium is adequate, it is often not true in developing countries where numerous pregnancies and a poor diet can lead to bone weakness.

A relationship between caffeine and osteoporosis has been found by some but not all researchers. A recent study of postmenopausal women found that higher lifetime consumption of caffeinated coffee was associated with lower bone density; however, this effect was not seen in coffee drinkers who also drank at least one glass of milk daily. Caffeine is found in coffee, tea, colas and other soft drinks, and some medicines. Since caffeine in large amounts can also cause chronic anxiety, disturbed sleep, and possibly to breast cysts, it is best to use it sparingly. Many heavy coffee drinkers are also smokers; these habits tend to be linked. Suggestions for quitting are discussed in Chapters 15 and 17.

Drinking large amounts of carbonated beverages, such as colas and other soft drinks, may be a risk factor for osteoporosis. Two recent studies showed that teenage girls and former college athletes over age 40 were both at increased risk of fracture if they consumed carbonated beverages. The former athletes drank an average of 50 gallons a year of soft drinks, which is close to the national average of 40 gallons a year! Phosphoric acid in such drinks, especially in colas, is under investigation as a cause of bone weakness.

MEDICATIONS TO PREVENT AND TREAT OSTEOPOROSIS

Osteoporosis can often be prevented and treated by estrogen; this hormone is very effective in halting the process of bone thinning and promoting bone strength. Numerous studies have shown a 30-50% reduction in bone fractures among women taking estrogen tablets, and many doctors regard this medication as an important answer to the problem of bone loss with aging. However, the effects of estrogen on bone rapidly decrease after the hormone is stopped, and the average age of hip fracture is 80. Taking estrogen for 5 or 10 years at menopause will probably not give bone protection 25 years later; it is necessary to stay on the hormone for many years to get its full benefits. For this reason, doctors are considering the following strategies for using estrogen to prevent hip fractures: 1) advise estrogen for women at the time of menopause and advise them to stay on it throughout life, 2) advise estrogen for those women who sustain an osteoporotic fracture, at the time of the fracture, thereby targeting the people at maximum risk of further fractures, or 3) start estrogen around age 65 and continue it for life, thereby ensuring that women are taking it in their most vulnerable years for hip fracture. Some women will be happy with the first option and others may decide on the second or third.

Women (and men) generally lose height with aging, due to thinning of their vertebrae and the disks between them, and due to postural changes. Studies of estrogen use have not yet shown that it has a significant effect in preventing this loss.

Women who have not had a hysterectomy need to take progesterone when they take estrogen, to prevent uterine cancer (see Chapter 10). Progesterone as well as estrogen helps to

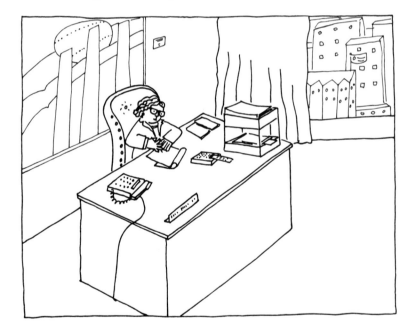

Janice, at 53, felt more secure after starting estrogen tablets to increase her bone strength. At 52 she had tripped on the street and fractured her ankle. The year before she broke her wrist when she fell on her stairs. Slim and small, Janice had followed a high-protein reducing diet for years. She had difficulty digesting milk products. She had a sedentary job in a bank and rarely exercised beyond doing housework. She was happy to take estrogen pills; they seemed the easiest solution and they also ended her hot flashes.

prevent bone loss, although its effectiveness against osteoporosis has not been studied as extensively as estrogen. Some women do not like the side effects of fatigue that can occur with progesterone, and others feel well with it. More study is urgently needed on the benefits and possible risks of various types of progesterone taken with or without estrogen for long periods of time.

Several new therapies for the prevention and treatment of osteoporosis are available, such as the bisphosphonates, calcitonin, and vitamin D analogs. These new medications do not contain estrogen, and may be helpful for women who need to seek an alternative. The bisphosphonates are medications that look like very good prospects for osteoporosis prevention and

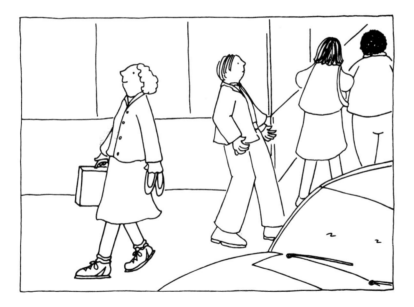

Ruth knew that she did not want to take hormones after menopause. She always tried to find natural remedies for physical problems and was not a believer in pills. She was determined to see menopause as a natural part of life, and not get upset by it. When her chiropractor told her she needed more exercise she joined a gym and began walking to and from work in tennis shoes. He also suggested that she chew mint-flavored calcium tablets after meals. She did some reading on menopause and felt secure in her decision to let nature take its course.

treatment. Alendronate (marketed as Fosamax) is currently the most promising of these medications. It appears to be quite effective in increasing bone density in the spine and the hip. Calcitonin, a hormone from the thyroid gland, acts to strengthen bone; it is taken by injection or by intranasal spray. It is often used after an osteoporotic fracture to reduce bone pain. Calcitonin has been extensively used in southern Europe and Japan; it is also available in the United States but is not widely used here. Calcitriol, a prescription drug, is the active form of vitamin D in the human body. Up to now it has been mainly used by people with severe kidney disease, who cannot produce their own activated vitamin D. Recent studies have shown that Calcitriol may be an effective medication for the prevention and treatment of osteoporosis. However, overdoses of Calcitriol can cause calcium-containing kidney stones, so its use must be carefully monitored. Other new medications, such as parathyroid hormone and ipriflavone (closely related to the soybean; see Chapter 15) are under study. More research is needed on all these treatments, but it is felt that they will provide an alternative for women at risk for osteoporosis who do not want to take estrogen.

This has been a complex chapter because of the many factors that influence bone strength. In summary, some people are more at risk than others for fractures due to osteoporosis. As the table on page 66 shows, the woman most at risk is White, thin, with a family history of fractures with aging, and an early menopause. These genetic risks are greatly increased if she smokes, drinks heavily, does not exercise, and eats a diet high in protein and salt and low in calcium. Conversely, women of any genetic background can greatly decrease their risk of fractures with aging by not smoking, exercising daily, eating lots of vegetables and calcium-rich foods, taking calcium supplements with vitamin D, and minimizing meat, salt, and caffeine in their diets. A bone-density study may help a woman understand her personal risk for osteoporosis. Estrogen and progesterone can be taken after menopause to preserve bone strength. These or other medications should be considered by those women most at risk for fractures. Everyone should eat healthily and find an enjoyable way to move.

Hormones and Psychology: Is Menopause a Time of Emotional Imbalance?

8

Popular mythology depicts the menopausal woman as going a little off her rocker. Are there special psychological risks for menopausal women? Are they more prone to depression, anxiety, irritability, and a general inability to cope?

If a woman in her late 40s gets angry or cries, her emotion is often blamed on "the change of life," just as in her 30s it was blamed on her periods or pregnancy. This kind of thinking can make women feel helpless, at the mercy of their hormones. It often prevents them from examining the factors in their relationships, families, or jobs that may well cause anger or depression.

*The group was talking about their emotional responses to menopause.
"Menopause has been really a hard time for me," said Sally. "I feel much
more vulnerable and get depressed easily. I cry when my daughter leaves*

home or if my boss is unreasonable." "Listen, Sally," said Petra, "you're facing the classic midlife crisis in my opinion. You'll be living alone when your daughter gets married and if your boss fires you, you're sunk!" "It's too bad it all happens at once," answered Sally. "I have a hard time coping with hot flashes, my boss, and my daughter's leaving." "Something similar happened to me," said Alice. "Then I moved into a house with some friends and it got better. I wasn't lonely and my expenses went way down. Actually I feel happier than I have in years—and I'm going through menopause, too."

It is important to attempt to identify the issues—do the end of ovulation and the drop of hormone levels at menopause create a psychological imbalance in some women, triggering depression, anxiety, or mood swings? Or is it the symptoms of menopause, especially the insomnia many women have, that make them chronically tired and edgy? Or maybe the real problem is

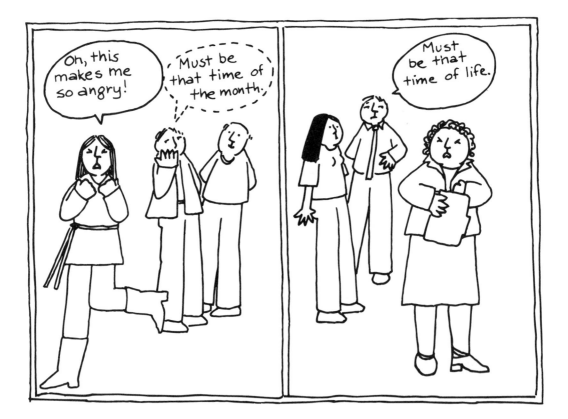

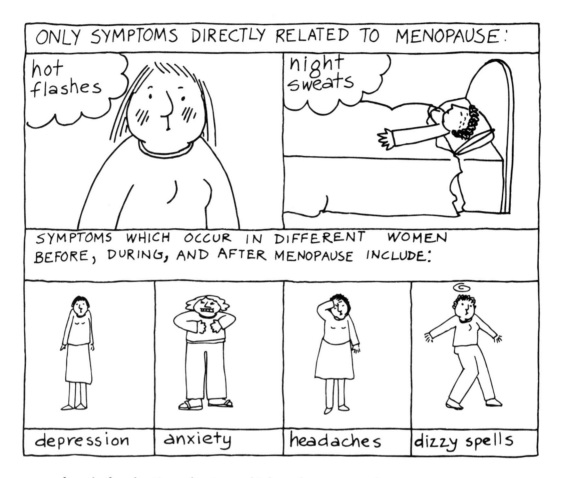

our culture's devaluation of aging, which makes women fear that their husbands or partners will leave them, or they will lose their job and not find another one. All of these factors can play a role in our psychology.

Serious emotional illness does not reach a peak as women go through menopause; in fact, severe depression and anxiety occur more often to women in their 30s than between 45 and 55. Other symptoms, such as mood swings, headaches or dizzy spells, occur in some women before, during, and after menopause, without a peak at any specific age. Moreover, these symptoms tend to occur together; some women experience many such problems, while others have very few.

But what about women who do feel anxious or depressed in their menopausal years? What are some typical problems they face, and what solutions are available?

CULTURAL FACTORS

In our society women have been judged by their physical appearance more than anything else. The emphasis we place on beauty, fashion, figure, and youth makes it difficult for some women to value themselves as they become middle aged. This is especially true for those who used their glamour and sexiness to attract men and enhance their sense of self-esteem. Many midlife women complain that they have become "invisible"—they no longer receive the attention they once enjoyed at social gatherings, and men seem to avoid them or look past them. It is especially devastating if a husband or lover leaves a woman for a younger partner. Even without this problem, a menopausal woman may become upset over vaginal dryness and pain with intercourse, feeling she is inadequate or invalidated as a sexual partner. She may feel that the end of her fertility means the end of her sexuality, and no longer view herself as a desirable person. She may consider hot flashes an embarrassing, visible sign of aging.

Feelings of depression and anxiety are understandable in these circumstances. However, not all women react to aging with depression despite the cultural pressures that reward youthful female beauty and sexiness. Women who value themselves in their work, their avocations, or as friends or family members, have an easier time adjusting to the waning of youth. They may see menopause as a welcome end to menstrual periods, and accept its bodily changes as normal. They go through the same hormonal process as the woman who becomes distraught, but they interpret it differently. Self-esteem is the key here—finding ways to value yourself as a person beyond your appearance. Support groups and psychotherapy can be very helpful in building a new sense of your worth.

When children leave home for jobs, college, or marriage, some mothers have problems with this loss which they may blame on menopause. Actually, this change can occur when a women is in her 30s or her 60s, depending on when the youngest child leaves home. And despite all the mythology about the "empty nest," most parents feel quite positive about their children's maturity. Some women, however, do feel they have lost a major reason for existence—this is especially true of women who have focused their energies primarily on their children. Feelings of anxiety and depression about the loss of the mother role can be very painful. So can feelings of guilt about parenting, if children's lives are disturbed by illness, drugs, unwanted pregnancy, or failure in school or work.

If the woman's anxieties are blamed on menopause, solutions are often sought in hormones or a tranquilizer and the real issue is left untouched. It is important for such women to reexamine what they want to do with their lives beyond mothering. They need to find new ways to express themselves which will raise their self-esteem, by going back to school, making new friends, getting a volunteer or paying job, or becoming politically active in an important cause. A counselor or a woman's group can be more valuable than a pill.

Some women become mothers in their late 30s or 40s, and go through menopause when their children are toddlers, preadolescents, or in the throes of puberty. This can be really taxing, because raising children takes such physical energy and steady purpose, and menopause is a time when many women crave time for themselves, to rethink their life's meanings. Children do not usually give you this opportunity! It is important for older mothers to have a partner who really shares the tasks of housework and parenting. If you have the means to do so, find extra childcare that enables you to spend a few hours a week by yourself—walking, learning something new, writing in a journal, or doing what calls to you. If possible, find other older parents for friendship, discussions and support.

Women who have interesting jobs, steady incomes, a sense of purpose, or things to do usually report fewer problems with menopause. Conversely, women without as many options, in unskilled or poorly paid jobs, often view menopause as more difficult. They may have less information about the physical symptoms of menopause and react to them with more anxiety. Other unrelated illnesses may exist which compound the problem. Medical care providers usually handle health problems with surgery, medicines, or tranquilizers, but may not have time to give the information and counseling that is needed to combat fears and years of negative stereotypes. Books, videos, talks and support groups play an important role here—fortunately in recent years, menopause has "come out of the closet," and we can talk about it more openly. This is enormously helpful to women.

Cultural anthropologists who look at women's roles in various societies believe that the social context of our lives determines our reactions to aging. In our culture, the emphasis on youth and the nuclear family structure can make menopause a lonely time for women. In many other cultures, aging increases the status, power, and freedom that women experience; the menopausal years bring recognition and leadership roles in the extended family, ceremonies, and commerce. Freedom from sexual taboos allows women to travel more easily. Postmenopausal women are able to cultivate the more assertive side of their nature. Some of this can be seen in our own society if we look at older women who learn new skills, return to school, go into politics, or excel in their professions. The stereotype of the menopausal woman is changing, and each one of us is part of that change.

When I give talks on menopause to groups of women, I like to hold a "shouting out" session when people say what it is they really want to do but have never had the time to begin. The atmosphere becomes infectious with emerging ambition. It is as valid to mention a tiny step as a huge one. Plant a garden, start to paint, climb in the Rockies, play the saxophone, go back to school, start a small business, learn to speak Spanish, find a new lover, run for the school board—it is obvious as women call out their wishes that this is a time for new beginnings. I love hearing these ambitions, because I know that many menopausal women are revitalized by carrying them out, one step at a time. If you have some ideas of your own, I advise you to give yourself the time to explore them. If you feel stuck about making such a choice, you may want to try free writing for 10 or 15 minutes a day—write whatever comes to you without stopping —no punctuation, no spelling worries—just keep your pen moving. If you don't like to write, try keeping an art journal, shouting out by yourself in the car, or talking into a tape recorder. Several books on these techniques are mentioned in the last chapter, *Suggestions for Further Reading*. If your focus is self-understanding, you will probably have some good ideas within a few weeks.

HORMONAL FACTORS

The hormones from our ovaries—mainly estrogen, progesterone and testosterone—play an important role in shaping our

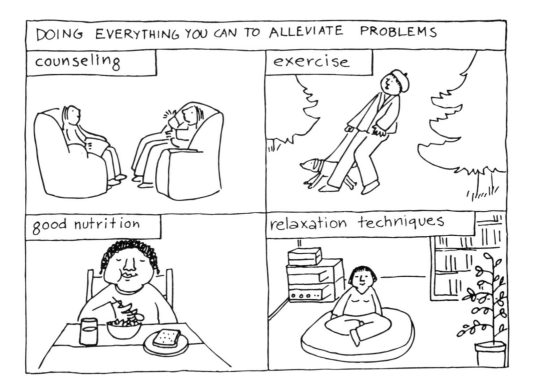

feelings and behavior. This is obvious in adolescence, when girls (and boys) begin to act wild and rebellious. Adults usually look knowingly at each other and say "hormones." What happens in menopause is more subtle, as our behavior patterns are more formed at this time. There is a period of readjustment, as estrogen levels no longer fluctuate with the menstrual cycle, but fall (slowly or quickly) to a steady, low level. Progesterone is virtually absent when ovulation no longer occurs. Testosterone is still secreted by the ovaries, though at lower levels than before. Nevertheless, testosterone may be relatively more dominant in postmenopausal women when their estrogen levels are low. This explains why older women may note more facial hair growth, and develop more assertive personalities! It has often been observed that the aging process helps women develop their "masculine" side, while men get in touch with their inner woman and become more nurturing and less competitive

The changes in hormone output throughout a woman's life affect each person differently. Some women notice marked changes in mood before each menstrual period, or become very depressed after childbirth, and some experience strong mood swings at menopause. Other women go through the menopausal transition without problems, and a few women note that it is a time of great well-being. We do not know if a woman who had premenstrual tension is at greater risk of problems with menopause—this should not automatically be assumed. It does appear that women who have had depressions earlier in life are most susceptible to depression in menopause.

Mood states are currently being studied from a biochemical perspective. The brain produces certain compounds (called neurotransmitters) that make us feel contented and euphoric, in response to exercise, food, love, meditation, touch, music, and other positive stimuli. Other compounds in the brain can make us irritable, anxious or depressed; these may be produced in response to overwork, boredom, frightening events, lack of sleep, drug or alcohol withdrawal, too little food, isolation and other unpleasant happenings. There is a complex interaction between our hormones and neurotransmitters, and both affect our states of mind. When estrogen levels fall at menopause, there is an accompanying fall in beta-endorphin levels in the brain. Since beta-endorphins are neurotransmitters associated with feelings of well-being, this shift may trigger depression or anxiety in some susceptible people. However, there are things you can do to enhance the creation of the "feel-good" neurotransmitters, such as sharing food with friends, finding an enjoyable form of exercise, getting a massage, listening to music, or whatever else works for you!

Studies have been done to evaluate the influence of hormone replacement on the mental and emotional states of menopausal women. Estrogen helps many women feel more cheerful and self-confident, but it is not helpful with major depressions or psychoses. A few women, on the other hand, feel emotionally uncomfortable on hormones, responding with anxiety or depression. When a progestin is taken, women may feel slightly more tired or irritable, as if they were experiencing some premenstrual tension.

It is hard to sort out the reasons for subtle shifts in our moods. Clearly our psychology, our outlook on life, is affected by the world around us and by our inner biology. The interactions among all these factors are so intimate that it is artificial to try to separate them. During the menopausal years the body goes through a major transition which is experienced differently by every woman, depending on her general health, her body awareness, and the rapidity of her hormone drop. Her psychological reaction to this transitional phase will be determined by both her biochemistry and her outer circumstances. Each affects the other—inner and outer worlds are inseparable, and in constant interaction.

Psychologists once proclaimed "biology is destiny"— meaning women were bound to go through certain predictable physical and emotional stages because of their reproductive systems. A more balanced viewpoint is that biology is only a part of destiny, along with the social environment in which we live. Moreover, as we understand this riddle we can direct at least some of our destiny by choosing to enhance our health and self-esteem.

Women reading this chapter may apply it individually according to their own experiences. Some will be pleased to discover that they need not become depressed or "go crazy" just because their periods stop. They need not experience the "raging imbalance of hormones" they have heard about. Other readers may feel that their emotional symptoms are intimately tied to their menopause, and will find relief in the knowledge that hormones can affect mood and emotions.

Menopausal women with physical or psychological problems are frequently given potent medications instead of the information and counseling they may need. Tranquilizers and sleeping pills generally belong to the family of drugs known as benzodiazepines. These drugs are chemically related to Valium; they are powerful, effective for sleep, but also addicting. In my experience as a doctor, long-term use (over 2 weeks for many people) can lead to unpleasant side effects and withdrawal symptoms. Sometimes withdrawal is so difficult it requires the

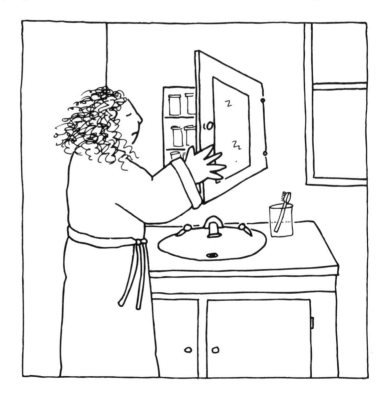

short-term use of phenobarbital. To avoid addiction, avoid tranquilizers and sleeping pills as much as possible, and do not use them for more than a few days at a time.

Antidepressants can be very effective for major depressions, but since they have side effects it is best to see a skilled psychiatrist to determine the best drug to use. Simultaneous counseling, with your psychiatrist or another counselor, may help shorten the time that antidepressants are needed.

Some women may want to take estrogen therapy for their physical and psychological symptoms. They should read Chapter 10 on the pros and cons of hormone therapy, and evaluate their response to the medicine with understanding.

Try making a list of all the natural methods you have found that put you in a better mood. Some people write their troubles in a journal and are able to understand and transcend them; some play the piano or learn to paint; some cook dinner for friends. Walking in nature, dancing and moving to music, relaxation techniques involving deep, slow abdominal breathing, massage, and good nutrition work for almost everyone—by changing brain chemistry towards balance and harmony. Sometimes what women need above all is to find—or establish—a self-help group of other midlife women, to develop more positive images of menopause and aging.

Gail had a very hectic job and had gotten into the habit of taking pills to calm down. Her internist gave her diuretics and tranquilizers. Her orthopedist gave her muscle relaxants. She took over-the-counter antihistamines and diet pills. She drank a fair amount of coffee throughout the day and alcohol at night to calm down. One day as Gail stood in front of her medicine cabinet she knew something was wrong. She felt terrible inside, shaky and weak. She realized that she never allowed herself to feel the normal state of her body—she was always taking something to alter it. Her medicine cabinet became a blur of yellow, orange, green, and white pills. "I'm going to stop all these drugs," she heard herself say. Gail had a very uncomfortable time of it, and had to take a leave of absence from work, but she did manage to quit taking all pills. She found that acupuncture helped her withdrawal problems, as did a self-help group. Now she just has a hectic job, but no drug problem. "I like knowing what my body is going through," said Gail. "I'd rather have an anxious hour than be in a chemical fog."

When Periods Stop Before 40   9

*J*ill's periods became very light and far apart when she was 30. The
next year they disappeared entirely and she began having hot flashes.
She had been hoping to get pregnant as soon as her recycled paper
business took off, so menopause was a really unpleasant surprise. Jill went
to a gynecologist who did some tests and told her she had a genetic
problem that had caused a smaller number of egg cells in her ovaries. He
also told her she could go to a big medical center in the state capital and
attempt pregnancy with an egg donated by another woman, but fertilized
by her husband's sperm. Jill and her husband were shocked by this news.
They had no health insurance, and could not afford the egg donation
treatment. Jill felt more like her old self when she took the hormones that
her doctor prescribed. After a year of thinking it over, she and her husband
decided to adopt a baby.

Menopause is considered premature if it occurs before the age of 40, and early if it comes between 40 and 45. Surgical removal of the uterus and ovaries is a common reason for premature menopause, and occasionally a woman goes into natural menopause before 40. Women who undergo cancer chemotherapy frequently experience menopausal symptoms during and after treatment. Younger women are more likely to regain their periods after chemotherapy, although menopause may occur earlier than it normally would have. Women over 40 often go directly into menopause as a result of chemotherapy. This chapter will look at premature menopause, discuss the problems of this condition, and make recommendations for preserving health and sexuality despite the cessation of periods.

CONDITIONS THAT ARE NOT PREMATURE MENOPAUSE

When a woman in her 20s or 30s stops having menstrual periods there may be many reasons for it. Pregnancy, stress, or illness are common causes, and weight loss, prolonged strenuous exercise, or excessive weight gain can also play a role. Stopping the birth-control pill may cause periods to cease for a year or more. Occasionally an excess of prolactin, the milk-promoting hormone of the pituitary, interrupts periods and causes milky fluid in the nipples. Phenothiazine drugs (Thorazine® and others) and related medicines prescribed for severe emotional illness produce similar results.

Each of these conditions—none of which is premature menopause—needs to be considered when a woman's periods prematurely stop. Blood tests to diagnose premature menopause mainly focus on two hormones from the pituitary gland which stimulate the ovary to ovulate; they're called follicle-stimulating hormone (FSH) and luteinizing hormone (LH). When these hormones are low, the ovaries are temporarily at rest, but the woman is not menopausal. The pituitary gland and the ovaries will generally resume their activity when a woman's general health, emotional well-being, or hormone

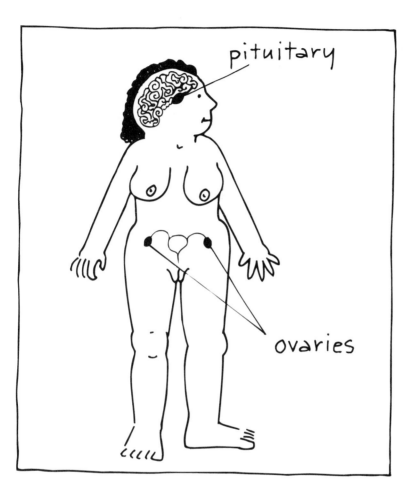

balance improves; the pituitary will put out more FSH and LH, the ovaries will be stimulated, and ovulation and menstruation will occur.

WHAT IS PREMATURE MENOPAUSE?

Sometimes the levels of FSH and LH are found to be very high. The ovaries are bombarded by stimuli but do not respond with ovulation, because the areas in the ovaries which produce egg cells and estrogenic hormones are scarce and nonfunctional.

This is premature menopause. Sometimes there is a genetic basis for this rare condition—the cells in the ovaries were programmed from birth to function for a shorter time because they were few in number or because of an abnormal gene. Another reason for premature menopause is that the woman develops antibodies to various glands in her body, such as her ovaries or her thyroid gland, thereby blocking glandular function. If you have premature menopause you should have blood tests to check for such antibodies, for while there is no good treatment as yet for this problem, replacement hormones often make you feel more normal.

When premature menopause occurs in a woman's 30s, she usually gets hot flashes in the same way older women do. If it occurs even earlier, her symptoms may be less noticeable. Some young women have menstrual periods for only a few years—and they never experience hot flashes. The current explanation for this is that these women have never become accustomed to a high estrogen level, so they do not react to its withdrawal (see Chapter 4).

PREGNANCY AND PREMATURE MENOPAUSE

Premature menopause can be extremely disappointing to the woman who wants to become pregnant. However, some women with a naturally occurring early menopause do conceive after hormone treatment or other new techniques in infertility treatment, including the donation of an egg from another woman. If you want to get pregnant, consult a gynecologist who specializes in infertility, or find the nearest center dealing with assisted reproductive techniques. There is a national organization of women with infertility problems, with many local chapters, support groups and the latest information. Contact *Resolve*, 1310 Broadway, Somerville, MA 02144-1731, telephone: 617-623-1156. If pregnancy is not possible for you, you may want to consider adopting a baby. An excellent book on adoption is included in *Suggestions for Further Reading* at the end of this book.

EARLY MENOPAUSE FROM CANCER CHEMOTHERAPY

When women in their reproductive years are given chemotherapy for breast or other cancers, they frequently lose their periods and develop menopausal symptoms. Younger women may regain their periods and fertility when the chemotherapy is over, but women over 35 or 40 often stay in menopause. If your cancer was not related to estrogen—for example, colon cancer or Hodgkin's disease—you will usually be given hormone therapy for the early menopause. Breast cancer patients, however, are advised not to use estrogen (although a few studies are underway on such treatment). Premenopausal breast cancer patients are told to expect hot flashes and a cessation of menstrual periods as a result of chemotherapy. They are often not told that they may also have a considerable and long-lasting problem with their sexuality, due to vaginal dryness and a loss of sex drive. Chemotherapy drugs such as Cytoxan, methotrexate, 5-FU and Adriamycin are more likely to cause sexual problems than tamoxifen (Nolvadex). It is important to note that not all women experience loss of sex drive with cancer chemotherapy. Small amounts of 1% testosterone cream applied to the clitoris may prove helpful with this problem—this should be discussed with your oncologist. See Chapter 4 for suggestions on how to deal with hot flashes; Chapters 14 and 15 on exercise and nutrition are also very important if you have had cancer.

EARLY MENOPAUSE FROM SURGERY

Surgically induced early menopause is quite common in the United States today. Some women enter menopause earlier after a hysterectomy even when their ovaries are retained, for reasons that are not completely understood. Surgery may disrupt the blood supply to the ovaries; another theory is that substances called prostaglandins secreted by the uterus may help with the cycle of ovulation. When the uterus is removed, ovulation may cease earlier than usual. Some women have

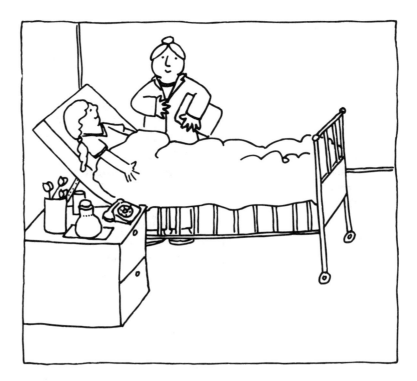

their ovaries removed at the time of a hysterectomy, even if the ovaries appear normal. This practice is diminishing, but many gynecologists believe that the 1% risk of ovarian cancer warrants the removal of healthy ovaries if the woman is over a certain age, say 40 or 45. The argument against this view, and in favor of retaining the ovaries whenever possible, is discussed in Chapter 3. This crucial point requires open discussion with the doctor before pelvic surgery, so you can make informed choices.

On the other hand, sometimes removing both ovaries is absolutely essential; overwhelming infection, tumors, cancer, severe endometriosis, or debilitating pelvic pain from scar tissue may leave no other course.

When Carolyn was 30 she had to have her uterus and both ovaries removed because of severe endometriosis. She was relieved to be without pain, but very sad to lose her fertility. Carolyn felt angry and cheated by her fate. She was given estrogen to prevent the symptoms of premature menopause, but she sometimes wondered if she should trust her doctor's prescription. At one point a friend persuaded her to stop taking the estrogen and try megavitamins and herbal capsules, but she developed severe hot flashes and vaginal dryness whenever she did so. Ultimately she resolved to stay on estrogen until her late 40s, and then taper the dose a bit. With time and counseling she regained a positive outlook, and pursued a career as a health professional. Later she married and adopted a baby.

If a young woman's ovaries are removed in surgery, she will undergo an abrupt premature menopause. She will not have the gradual decrease in estrogen experienced by women with natural menopause, so her symptoms may be more intense. Doctors routinely prescribe estrogen therapy at once, unless the surgery was done for a cancer promoted by estrogen.

What is the best advice for the woman with premature menopause? Should she take replacement hormones? What does she need to know in order to make a wise decision?

REPLACEMENT HORMONES

Copying nature as closely as possible has many advantages in this situation. The ovaries normally secrete estrogen, progesterone, and androgens (such as testosterone) until age 50, and androgens thereafter into old age. Some of these androgens are converted to estrogen in body fat. If you have had a premature menopause you can duplicate this situation by taking a moderate dose of estrogen until your mid-40s, and a lower dose thereafter. If you have retained your uterus you should take a progestin along with the estrogen, as explained in Chapter 10. These hormones will prevent hot flashes, vaginal dryness or soreness, and osteoporosis (see Chapter 7), which otherwise might begin earlier in life and cause fractures at a younger age.

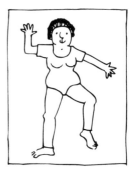

Many women feel well on these replacement hormones and find that their sex drive is satisfactory. However, some women with premature menopause are quite distressed by a lowering of their sexual responsiveness at an age when other women are reaching their peak. If estrogen does not restore sexual interest, doctors can prescribe a low dose of testosterone as a pill or as 1% testosterone cream to be applied to the clitoris every other day in small amounts. Since testosterone pills have some side effects, using testosterone cream may be the safest method (see Chapter 10).

Women whose ovaries are removed by surgery before their normal menopause run a higher risk of having a heart attack later on. The reason for this is believed to be that the body's estrogen alters the levels and types of blood fats in a healthy way. When the ovaries are removed this protection is missing, but replacement estrogen in pill form can produce a similar protective effect, as discussed in Chapter 10.

In deciding to take estrogen, women with premature menopause are helping to prevent discomfort and long-term problems of heart and bone disease (osteoporosis); at the same time the medication may cause some problems. No estrogen taken by mouth can exactly copy the complex ebb and flow of natural hormone secretions. The data on side effects from estrogen replacement are discussed in detail in the following chapter. Although most women with premature menopause do decide to take estrogen, some do not. For these women it is especially important to guard against osteoporosis and heart disease with exercise and good nutrition. You should exercise vigorously every day to keep your bones strong and promote cardiac fitness. You should not smoke or drink excess alcohol. You should eat a low-fat, high-calcium diet without too much salt or protein, to prevent osteoporosis. You would do well to consult a physician who is interested in preventive medicine, so you can monitor your bone strength and risk factors for heart disease.

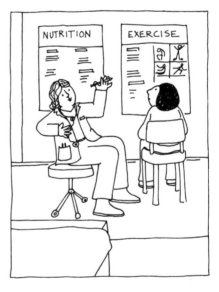

Hormone Replacement Therapy

10

No one ever told us we had to study our lives, make of our lives a study, as if learning natural history.

—Adrienne Rich

The women in the group were discussing hormones. "My doctor told me he prescribes them for almost all his patients," said Wendy. "He made me feel I'd be really negligent of my health if I didn't start estrogen. Then I talked to my mother, and she just laughed. She's been healthy as a horse without hormones, and she's straight as a broom at 75." "I don't know what to do," said Roberta. "My cholesterol is a little high, and there's a history of heart attack in my family. But my sister has breast cancer, so I'm really scared of taking hormones." "So quit the butter and cheese and join our walking group!" said Clara. "I've been telling you this for years and now maybe you'll listen." Finally Carol spoke up: "It's been really important for me to take estrogen. It's made me feel much better mentally and physically. And I'm so glad to be rid of hot flashes and be able to sleep through the night." "I'm glad there's finally some research on this question," said Clara. "It's been billions for outer space, pennies for inner."

Amazing advances in chemistry and pharmacology in our time have created many new choices for doctors and patients.

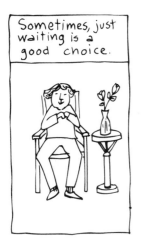

Sometimes, just waiting is a good choice.

Common discomforts and aging itself are no longer accepted as inevitable. Instead they are combated with medicines and procedures, some very helpful—and others potentially dangerous. We must all tackle the difficult chore of reasonably choosing among the possible therapies for our problems. Sometimes just waiting is a good choice, and sometimes treatment is necessary. The menopausal woman's choice about using hormones or not must be made carefully, because the therapy is relatively new; controversial in some ways, yet quite helpful to certain women. The benefits and risks of taking hormones—and not taking them—vary from person to person. In this chapter we will look at the pros, cons, and unknowns of hormone therapy in some detail. The following chapter summarizes the information more briefly, and provides a self-rating scale to help you make a careful decision, together with your doctor or nurse practitioner.

A LITTLE HISTORY

Since the beginnings of human evolution, women have gone through menopause without taking hormones. It's true that surviving to middle age used to be harder than it is now, but for centuries many people have lived to old age, women often

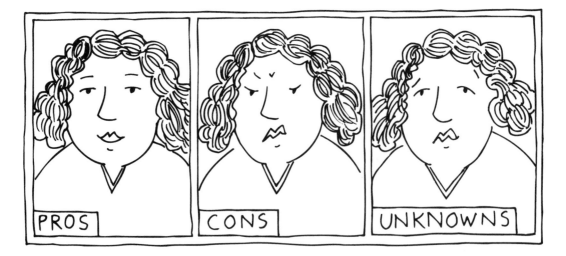

PROS   CONS   UNKNOWNS

outliving men. In places today where many women and men live to be 100—remote mountainous areas in Ecuador, Pakistan, or southern Russia—the use of estrogen therapy is certainly very low! Extreme longevity seems to depend not on any drug therapy, but on a favorable family history and a lifestyle characterized by exercise, moderate eating and drinking, and an optimistic attitude.

When estrogen was first isolated in the 1920s, it was used for women who had lost their ovaries through surgery, as well as for women with severe problems after natural menopause. However, its use was not widespread until the 1960s, when a book entitled *Feminine Forever*, by Robert Wilson, popularized estrogen use. Women wanted ERT (estrogen replacement therapy) because they were told they would age more slowly, look more attractive, and avoid the discomforts of menopause. Many doctors promoted ERT because it was a powerful and effective new treatment that provided an apparently quick answer to problems that were hard to deal with, like hot flashes, insomnia, vaginal soreness, midlife crises, and depression. While the drug does deal with the first three problems, it does not necessarily solve the social and psychological difficulties of the middle years. Helping a patient clarify such problems through counseling takes more time than the average doctor can spare, so prescriptions are often written as an alternative.

Another interested party in this use of estrogen has been the drug companies which manufacture the multitude of pills, patches, and creams designed for menopausal women. Thirty to forty million women in the United States today are postmenopausal. In some middle-class areas, more than half the postmenopausal women used ERT in 1975.

In the mid-1970s reports began to appear linking estrogen use in postmenopausal women to cancer of the uterus. Women were found to be about 5 times more likely to develop this cancer if they used estrogen replacement therapy. There was a rapid decline in the prescription of ERT after these reports, and this decline lasted several years. Recently, however, studies have shown that taking a progestin along with estrogen protects women quite effectively against uterine cancer. As this reassuring news became known, doctors began to prescribe postmenopausal hormones again. The use of a progestin along with estrogen is known as HRT, for "hormone replacement therapy."

The widespread use of postmenopausal hormones in western society today has several justifications. It is a response to the great increase in women's longevity in this century, in which the average life span has increased from 60 to 80 years. Older women's problems with broken bones can be substantially decreased with hormone use. Their tendency to develop heart disease and heart attack can also be diminished by estrogen. On the other hand, never before in human history has a large group of aging women taken medicines to prolong the youthful hormonal state of the reproductive years into the 50s and 60s and beyond. This alteration of the natural plan for the human body may have both benefits and risks, which need to be uncovered by painstaking study. Some questions about the effects of HRT are being answered; some are still being debated. What are the types of currently available hormones and their advantages and disadvantages?

ESTROGEN: TYPES AND METHODS OF USE

Estrogens that occur naturally in people are of three types: estrone, estradiol, and estriol. Estradiol is the principal estrogen naturally present in women before menopause; estrone is the main estrogen present after menopause. Estrone and estradiol are very similar and each can be converted into the other within the body. Estriol is a weak estrogen created by the placenta and the breakdown of other estrogens in the body. It is currently used very little in the U.S., but is used as a pill and vaginal cream in Europe.

Most estrogen tablets currently on the market in the U.S. are composed of various forms of estrone or estradiol. Estrace, Estraderm, Ogen and Ortho-Est closely resemble or are identical to human estrogens. Premarin, a commonly prescribed estrogen, is a mixture of estrone, estradiol and various types of horse estrogen, since it is derived from pregnant mares' urine.

The relative advantages of different types of estrogen have not been thoroughly studied.

In my opinion, women should not take any estrogen that is combined with a tranquilizer, such as PMB, which contains meprobamate. Meprobamate causes sedation and can be habit-forming. Experts believe that tranquilizers should be used only when absolutely necessary for anxiety, and never given with a drug designed for daily administration. Menopausal women should avoid taking the so-called nonsteroidal estrogens, such as DES (diethylstilbestrol) or TACE, because of the association of these drugs with vaginal cancer in the female children of women who took the medicines in pregnancy. The nonsteroidal estrogens are chemically less similar to natural estrogens, and need further safety evaluation.

Estrogen is also available in adhesive patches, known as Estraderm, or Climara, which are applied to the skin of the abdomen or thigh. The hormone is gradually and evenly absorbed through the skin. The patches are changed once or twice a week, but the woman is free to bathe or swim at any time. There may be significant advantages and disadvantages to using estrogen by skin patch compared to the usual tablet form. The patch gives an even blood level of estrogen throughout the day, while tablets taken by mouth give higher blood levels initially followed by a dropping off before the next pill is taken. The even absorption of estrogen through the skin helps some women with menopausal symptoms. When estrogen is taken by tablet it is absorbed through the intestinal tract and travels immediately to the liver, where it stimulates the production of a substance which causes high blood pressure in some individuals. Since estrogen by skin patch avoids this step it seems to be preferable for women prone to blood-pressure problems. On the other hand, there is concern that estrogen absorbed through the skin may not have the same favorable effect on blood cholesterol that is found with oral tablets. The patch causes an itchy skin rash in some users, and may not be as well absorbed if you sweat a good deal.

Estraderm patches come in three strengths, .025 mg, .05 mg and .1 mg. The lowest dose, .025 mg, is available in Europe and Canada but not in the U.S. Climara patches come in .05 and .1 mg dosages.

Table of Commonly Prescribed Estrogens

Brand Name	Generic Name	Tablet Strength
Climara	estradiol	.05 mg, .1 mg patch
Estrace	estradiol	.5 mg,* 1 mg,* 2 mg*
Estraderm	estradiol	.05 mg, .1 mg patch
Ogen	estropipate (estrone)	.625 mg,* 1.25 mg,* 2.5 mg,* 5 mg*
Ortho-EST	estropipate (estrone)	.625 mg,* 1.25 mg,*
Menest	estrone	.3 mg, .625mg, 1.25mg, 2.5mg
Premarin	conjugated estrogens	.3 mg, .625 mg, .9 mg, 1.25 mg, 2.5 mg
Premarin with methyltestosterone	conjugated estrogens (E) methyltestosterone (T)	.625 mg E + 5 mg T 1.25 mg E + 10 mg T
Estratest	esterified estrogens (E) methyltestosterone (T)	.625 mg E + 1.25 mg T 1.25 mg E + 2.5 mg T

When this mark (*) follows a dose it means the tablet is scored and can easily be divided in half.

USE OF A PROGESTIN WITH ESTROGEN

Estrogen used alone after menopause has been associated with an increased risk of uterine cancer. This risk can be greatly reduced or eliminated by adding a progestin tablet daily to the last 10 to 14 days of the cycle. Progestins are compounds similar to progesterone, normally secreted by the ovaries after ovulation and in pregnancy. It is extremely important that any woman who still has her uterus use one of the following schedules if she wishes to take HRT.

Schedule 1: She should take an estrogen pill from the 1st to the 25th day of the month. She should also take a progestin from the 14th to the 25th day. Then she should stop taking both tablets for 5 or 6 days, and at this point she will usually have some bleeding. The progestin tablet has the effect of allowing the uterine lining to be evenly shed when all hormones are stopped. If the lining is sloughed off this way every month, it is much less likely that it will become cancerous. Some doctors use a variation on this schedule, prescribing estrogen pills every day without stopping, and adding a progestin for 10 to 12 days each month. Bleeding should occur at the end of the progestin phase.

Schedule 2: She should take a low-dose progestin pill with each estrogen pill on a continuous basis. Alternatively she can take both pills for 5 days of each week and skip them both for 2 days. The main advantage of this method is the elimination of monthly periods, which many women appreciate. However, there is usually some irregular bleeding during the first few months on this schedule; it may take 6 to 12 months before all bleeding stops. A disadvantage for some women is that a progestin can give side effects of fatigue, irritability or increased appetite.

Adding a progestin to the estrogen cycle greatly reduces the risk of uterine cancer, but it can have disadvantages. Progestin compounds in the birth-control pill were found to cause changes in the body's use of starches and sugars similar to the changes of diabetes, and to alter blood fats in an unfavorable way. They were implicated, along with estrogen, in high blood pressure, heart disease, and stroke. The type of progestins used in birth-control pills are therefore not desirable for older women and in my opinion should not be used for long-term hormone replacement therapy. Norlutate, Norlutin, and Aygestin are examples of this type of progestin. Medroxyprogesterone acetate, marketed as Provera, Amen or Cycrin, is a safe progestin for the postmenopausal woman. Provera (Amen or Cycrin) is generally prescribed in a 5 or 10 mg dose when given for 10-14 days (Schedule 1, above) and in a 2.5 mg dose when given daily with estrogen (Schedule 2, above). Premphase (Schedule 1) and Prempro (Schedule 2) are products which have the estrogen Premarin packaged along with Provera, giving users the convenience of having their daily pills accessible in one packet, labeled by days of the week. The disadvantage is the greater cost of this packaging.

Many women do not have bothersome side effects from progestins, but some cannot tolerate them. If this is a problem for you, you can consider the following options. The safest variation is to ask your doctor to prescribe natural micronized progesterone, as described in the next paragraph. Alternatively, discuss with your doctor the safety of taking a 14-day course of a progestin every other month, or every third month. Have your uterine lining monitored for its thickness with vaginal ultrasound, or removed on a yearly basis with a thorough endometrial aspiration. These techniques have not been researched as much as regular progestin use for the prevention of uterine cancer, but they are being tried quite often today and more information should soon be available.

Natural progesterone, identical to the hormone made by the ovaries, was not used for many years because it was not absorbed when taken in pill form. Thanks to a new technique of decreasing the particle size of progesterone—micronization— and suspending it in oil, natural progesterone in pill form is now effective. A new type is designed to be dissolved under the tongue. Natural progesterone is in use in several European countries, but has not been approved by the FDA for use in the U.S. However, natural progesterone was recently used in a 3-year trial sponsored by the National Institutes of Health, in which it was compared to the progestin Provera for effects on cholesterol. Natural progesterone plus estrogen was found to be the most favorable combination of medications in terms of a favorable effect on cholesterol and minimal weight gain. As it has a short duration of action, natural progesterone must be taken 2 to 3 times daily, in 100-mg capsules. It is also available as rectal or vaginal suppositories, and in a form that is dissolved under the tongue. Natural progesterone is somewhat more expensive than the progestins that are usually prescribed. Its main side effect is sleepiness, which affects some but not all women. Doctors can order natural progesterone for their patients from a variety of mail-order pharmacies, and local pharmacies in some areas.

Creams said to contain natural progesterone from plant sources are sold in natural food stores, and have become quite popular for the alleviation of hot flashes. Many of these creams are not adequately labeled, so the user does not know how much progesterone they contain, or how much she may be absorbing. Such creams should not be used to balance estrogen for the prevention of uterine cancer—they may not be effective.

If the woman's uterus has been removed by surgery, she can take a few days off estrogen each month, but she need not take a progestin. Any woman who has a uterus, however, should take a progestin or natural micronized progesterone whenever she takes daily estrogen. This is taken to prevent an excessive buildup of the uterine lining, which occasionally leads to uterine cancer. The addition of a progestin is also a good idea for a woman who has taken estrogen alone in the past and is no longer taking it; a 10- to 14-day course of progestin will bring on a period if she has any significant thickness to her uterine lining. Uterine cancer can occur years after a woman has taken estrogen alone, without a progestin. Some doctors prescribe a progestin even if estrogen has never been taken, especially in women who seem to produce abundant natural estrogen after menopause. This occurs more often in women who have considerable body fat.

TESTOSTERONE USE

As explained in Chapter 3, the ovaries put out androgens (formerly called "male hormones") such as testosterone, throughout a woman's lifetime, although the amount produced falls at menopause. These hormones contribute to muscle strength, appetite, a sense of well-being and sex drive. Women who have both ovaries removed sometimes do not feel as energetic and sexual as they did before surgery, even with estrogen replacement, possibly because of their lower levels of testosterone. (This is variable, however, as some women do well on estrogen replacement alone; they are probably getting enough androgens from their adrenal glands.) In recent years some doctors have been prescribing oral testosterone along with estrogen for women whose ovaries have been removed, or for women after natural menopause who complain of lack of sex drive.

While these treatments are helpful in the short term, there may be risks with continued use. When testosterone is given as a pill, it is given in a form known as methyltestosterone. This is the type of testosterone found in Estratest and in Premarin with Methyltestosterone tablets, where it is combined with estrogen. Liver disease has been associated with the use of oral methyltestosterone—ranging from hepatitis due to accumulation of bile in the liver, to peliosis hepatis (a life-threatening accumulation of blood in the liver), to liver cancer. While these cases are rare, and generally involve higher doses given to men, the safety of low doses in women has not been carefully studied. Even though the above-named pills are on the market, the FDA has never approved the use of methyltestosterone for women. Methyltestosterone was once considered as an oral contraceptive for men, but was rejected by the World Health Organization because of the danger of liver problems. I find these facts a disturbing example of the prescription of drugs to women without adequate safety testing.

An injectable form of testosterone, known as testosterone enanthate or cypionate, has not been associated with liver disease. However, the amounts given in injections or implants can be higher than normal for a woman, and can cause a permanent lowering of the voice, hair growth on the face or balding at the temples. In addition, all forms of testosterone can have unfavorable effects on blood fat levels, by lowering the desirable HDL cholesterol fraction. This can be a problem for women with risk factors for heart disease.

A possible connection between testosterone in women and breast cancer is under investigation by some cancer researchers. Women have an enzyme in their fat cells known as aromatase, which converts testosterone to estrogen. The conversion of ovarian testosterone to estrogen in body fat is an important source of estrogen after menopause. The fat cells in our breasts, and cells in a majority of breast cancers, also contain the enzyme aromatase, and thereby produce estrogen. Both estrogen and testosterone have been shown to stimulate breast cancer cell division in the laboratory.

Several European studies have shown that women with breast cancer have a higher chance of relapse after surgery if they have higher levels of testosterone in their blood and urine. In addition, a study from the Danish Cancer Registry showed that Danish women taking a combination of estrogen and testosterone had a higher risk of breast cancer than women using estrogen alone, or estrogen and a progestin. I feel that any relationship between breast cancer and testosterone supplements is suggestive rather than conclusive at this point, and deserves a good deal of further study. However, until we know more about the long-term effects of using this hormone, I feel that doctors and women should be very cautious about its use.

Despite these possible risks, there is a valid need for testosterone replacement in certain cases—women who have lost their sex drive due to ovarian removal or cancer chemotherapy can be extremely distressed. The safest way to use testosterone is probably to apply a small amount of 1% testosterone cream to the clitoris and surrounding area—a pea-sized dab of cream on the end of your finger is the amount to apply. The cream is used daily for 1 week and then 2 to 3 times a week as needed for sexual drive. This therapy often has good results with the least amount of systemic absorption. The cream must be prescribed by a doctor and made to order by a pharmacist. Research is needed on doses, absorption and blood levels of testosterone before and after this kind of topical use on and around the clitoris.

In addition, doctors and women patients should avoid ovarian removal unless it is really necessary. There are now alternative treatments which make it possible to avoid a hysterectomy in many (not all) cases, and women undergoing a hysterectomy can elect to retain their ovaries if these organs appear healthy. It is better for most women to rely on the low levels of testosterone secreted by the ovary throughout life than to use supplemental products with potentially problematic side effects.

REASONS FOR TAKING POSTMENOPAUSAL ESTROGENS

Let's review the reasons women and their doctors favor using estrogens, and the dosages appropriate in each situation. Women under the age of 45 who have had an early menopause or a surgical menopause should review Chapter 9 before reading this section.

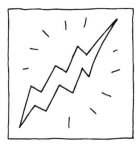

Hot flashes and insomnia

Estrogen will act rapidly to reduce these problems. The lowest dose that will prevent discomfort is the goal, and therefore women should keep a record of their hot flashes and start with the lowest dose of estrogen available. For some currently marketed products these doses are: Premarin .3 mg, Ortho-EST or Ogen .3 mg (obtained by dividing the .625 mg tablet), Menest .3mg, and Estrace .5 mg (obtained by dividing the 1 mg tablet). Since estrogen is best absorbed with some food in the stomach, take your tablet with a little bit of food. This is especially important for women taking the lowest possible doses.

Estrogen tablets are usually very effective in reducing hot flashes, night sweats and the accompanying insomnia that many women experience. It may take a few weeks of estrogen use before the full effect is noticed. However, these symptoms generally return when estrogen is stopped. Taking estrogen, therefore, does not cure hot flashes but it does postpone them until the time that HRT is stopped. Some women elect to take HRT indefinitely and thus may never have hot flashes. Other women take estrogen for temporary relief of hot flashes and then decide to stop it after a few months or a few years. Since the mechanisms involved in hot flashes are related to rapid decrease in estrogen levels (see Chapter 4), the best way to cease estrogen therapy is to taper off very slowly. The woman taking .625 mg of conjugated estrogen can switch to .3 mg daily for a month or two, then take this dose every other day, and finally stop it entirely. She should continue taking a progestin as well unless her uterus has been removed. Sometimes after a 3- to 6-month trial of this regimen, hot flashes will be lessened. If not, the woman can resume estrogen and repeat the tapering-off process when she is ready. Many women find they can cope with the problems of hot flashes when they gradually and slowly reduce the estrogen dose this way.

If estrogen cannot be used, some doctors use injectable or oral progestins alone to relieve hot flashes. These medications are not quite as effective as estrogen, but do help in many cases. See Chapter 4 for several other suggestions on how to minimize hot flashes.

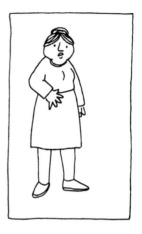

Vaginal soreness

Insertion of a penis, fingers, or a vaginal speculum can be uncomfortable or painful in postmenopausal women, because estrogen and androgen secretion from the ovaries has

Table of Estrogen and Testosterone Vaginal Creams

Brand Name	Generic Name	Strength	Comments
Ogen cream	estropipate (estrone)	1.5 mg per gram of cream	Use very small amount as explained in text, page 112.
Premarin cream	conjugated estrogens	.625 mg per gram of cream	
Estrace cream	estradiol	.1 mg per gram of cream	
Ortho Dienestrol cream	dienestrol		Dienestrol is a synthetic estrogen. Not enough is known about its effects and dosages; not recommended.
Estriol cream	estriol	.5 mg per gram	Available by prescription from some mail-order pharmacies; generic.
Testosterone cream	testosterone propionate	1% or 2% in vanishing cream base	Must be made by pharmacist; generic only.

decreased. One action of these hormones is to keep the vaginal lining cells thickened and resistant to friction. When hormone levels drop, this cellular layer becomes thinner, drier, and less elastic. The vagina is then more likely to be sore or irritated by penetration. This situation can be alleviated by estrogen tablets, the estrogen patch, or by the use of a low-dose estrogen cream. Many women decide to take estrogen because of its beneficial effects on their vagina and their sexual comfort. Other women go through menopause and beyond with very little vaginal discomfort, and do not need estrogen for this function.

One of the commonly used estrogen creams is Premarin cream. This comes with an applicator calibrated for 1 to 4 grams of cream; the dose frequently suggested is 2 to 4 grams daily or ½ to 1 applicator applied vaginally. As there is .625 mg of Premarin per gram of the cream, this dose would give a woman 1.25 to 2.5 mg of estrogen daily. The estrogen is rapidly absorbed from the vagina. In fact, estrogen cream in high doses can be stronger than pills, as hormones from the cream directly enter the blood stream and are not subject to the digestive process.

However, lower doses of estrogen cream than currently suggested by most doctors and drug companies are effective. I advise women to use ½ gram (⅛ of an applicator) of Premarin cream, which corresponds to a .3 mg Premarin tablet, or 1 gram of Estrace cream, which corresponds to ¹⁄₁₀ of a 1 mg Estrace tablet. The cream should be directed towards the sore area which is usually inside the inner vaginal lips right at the entrance to the vagina. Apply the cream to that area with the applicator or with a finger, being sure to get to the sorest point. After 5 to 10 days of such treatment, the problem of pain with penetration is usually resolved. Thereafter, most women then use the cream every 2 or 3 days. Do not use the cream right before sex; it is designed for vaginal treatment, not as a lubricant, and could affect your sexual partner.

One study suggested that after about a week of estrogen cream use with these very low doses, the vaginal cells seem to erect a partial barrier to the systemic absorption of estrogen, so that no increased blood levels of estrogen were found. More research is needed to clarify the systemic effects of the very low doses of cream required to relieve vaginal discomfort.

When such small doses are used, is there a risk of uterine cancer? Probably not; but to be safe, some doctors recommend the use of a progestin for 10 days after a few months of cream use, and every 6 months thereafter.

The use of these minimal doses of estrogen cream eliminates most of the pain of vaginal penetration. However, it does not restore as much vaginal lubrication as was present before menopause, so it's wise to use a lubricant during intercourse.

Testosterone cream is also effective in preventing vaginal soreness after menopause. It must be compounded by a pharmacist as 1% or 2% testosterone cream in a water-soluble base. It is used in the same way as estrogen cream: after a week or so of daily application, minimal amounts are effective twice weekly. It is thought to be safer than estrogen cream for women who have had breast cancer, but there are no studies on this point. Estriol cream, available from a few mail-order pharmacies, is also considered a better choice for women who have had breast cancer. Estriol is the weakest of the three forms of human estrogen; estriol cream is used in Europe to prevent vaginal and urinary tract infections in older women.

Osteoporosis—brittle bones

As Chapter 7 spells out, estrogen therapy retards the loss of calcium from bones after menopause. Since HRT results in a lower rate of hip and forearm fractures, doctors often suggest women most at risk of osteoporosis begin HRT at menopause and continue it for many years. Alternatively, women can start HRT if they develop osteoporosis, or at the age of 65, as discussed in Chapter 7.

The dose of HRT needed to prevent bone fractures probably varies from person to person. Most doctors are prescribing .625 mg of Premarin or Ogen, 1-2 mg of Estrace, or the .05 Estraderm patch, with a progestin taken daily or at the end of each cycle (if the uterus is present). Recent research suggests that a smaller dose, namely .5 mg of Estrace or .3 mg of Premarin, when combined with a calcium intake of 1,500 mg daily through the diet or supplements, is also protective against bone loss in most women. In the meantime, remember that all midlife women, including those on hormones, need to get daily exercise and an increased calcium intake to keep their bones strong.

Colon cancer prevention

Several recent studies have shown a significant decrease in colon cancer and deaths from this disease among women using hormone therapy. More research is needed to confirm these findings. Since colon cancer is a major problem for older women, this may turn out to be an important benefit of hormone use. Research has also shown that a high-fiber, low-fat diet, rich in vegetables and fruits, can help to prevent colon cancer. Calcium, vitamin D and exercise may also be protective.

Heart disease prevention

Heart disease is the major cause of death in women over the age of 65. When women who take estrogen after menopause are compared to those who do not, estrogen users are found to have about a 40-50% reduction in risk of fatal heart attack. This lower risk is seen in all groups of women, even those with the predisposing factors for heart disease—high blood pressure, high cholesterol levels, obesity, smoking, or a family history of early heart attack (before age 60). It is thought that estrogen confers these benefits by several mechanisms—by lowering total cholesterol levels and by enhancing the ability of blood vessels to dilate and permit more blood flow to the heart and other vital organs.

Estrogen has the same effects on blood cholesterol as a low-fat diet and exercise—it lowers the total cholesterol count and raises the high-density lipoprotein fraction of cholesterol known as HDL, which appears to protect blood vessels. Women who already have a total cholesterol under 200 and a high HDL level, who do not smoke or have high blood pressure, have little risk of heart attack provided they continue to exercise regularly and eat a low-fat diet. Estrogen replacement would not be as important to them as to other women with one or more risk factors mentioned above.

The progestins that women take along with estrogen to prevent uterine cancer can reduce some of the favorable effects of estrogen on the heart, but there is still a substantial net gain of protection compared to nonusers. Natural micronized progesterone has the least negative effect, followed by medroxyprogesterone acetate (Provera, Amen or Cycrin). Norethindrone (Norlutin, Norlutate or Aygestin) is felt to be less desirable for long-term use.

Women considering the use of postmenopausal hormones should understand these beneficial effects on the prevention of heart disease. Those with risk factors for this problem (outlined above) should talk to a doctor about the benefits of hormones in their case. Women without current risk factors who are not willing or able to exercise or eat a low-fat diet might also benefit from estrogen for long-term heart disease prevention.

There are several nonwestern societies in the world where death by heart attack is still quite rare. People eat a simple diet with few animal foods, and are physically active all their lives. It is difficult, but not impossible, to live this way in our modern world. All forms of moderate exercise are helpful, and many delicious foods can give you substantial protection, as explained in Chapters 14 and 15. A workable plan to lower your risk of heart disease without drugs is found in two books by Dean Ornish, MD—*Stress, Diet and Your Heart*, and *Dr. Dean Ornish's Program for Reversing Heart Disease*. Dr. Ornish prescribes a low-fat, vegetarian diet, daily walking, yoga and meditation, and group therapy to modify feelings of hostility and impatience which can cause blood vessels to go into spasm and reduce blood flow to the heart. All women and men in the second half of life can benefit from this advice.

Additionally, recent research suggests that women over age 50 may benefit from low-dose aspirin therapy (½ aspirin tablet every other day) for the prevention of heart attack. Talk to your doctor about this, especially if you have risk factors for heart disease. Taking a vitamin B complex and antioxidant vitamins such as E and beta carotene can also help, as explained in Chapter 16.

REASONS FOR NOT TAKING POSTMENOPAUSAL ESTROGEN

Cancer of the breast

Breast cancer, along with lung cancer, is the major cause of death today for women ages 40-65, and the rate at which it occurs is increasing. Recent studies have shown that the long-term use of postmenopausal hormones is probably one factor related to the occurrence of breast cancer. (Readers should know that scientists are still debating this subject—some discount the role of postmenopausal estrogen in promoting breast cancer.) The most comprehensive work on this subject comes from The Nurses' Health Study, in which 122,000 U.S. nurses have been followed since 1976 by investigators from Harvard Medical School. This study has shown that the risk of breast cancer and death from breast cancer goes up with long-term use of hormones—after 5 years of use there is about a 45% increase in risk. A 45% increase can be understood as follows: if 10 women out of a group of 100 would get breast cancer without using estrogen, 14-15 would contract the disease using it. This study also showed that age is a factor in the increased risk of breast cancer—women taking hormones at the age of 60 to 65, for example, appear to be more at risk than women between 50 and 55.

Estrogen and progesterone both seem to be implicated in this increased cancer risk. The addition of a progestin or progesterone is known to greatly reduce the risk of uterine cancer, but it does not similarly reduce the risk of breast cancer. For this reason, most doctors agree that women without a uterus should not take a progestin when they take estrogen.

There are other risk factors for breast cancer, unrelated to taking estrogen supplements. These include the finding of "fibroadenoma," "atypical hyperplasia" or "atypical proliferative cells" in a breast biopsy, not having borne children or having a first child late in life, being tall, and being overweight after menopause. The early onset of puberty or late onset of menopause may increase risk. A gene for breast cancer has been identified, and 5-10% of breast cancers have a family inheritance pattern. Women who were given DES (diethylstilbestrol) during pregnancy to prevent miscarriage show an increased risk of breast cancer beginning 20 years later. Some environmental pollutants, such as the breakdown products of plastics and DDT, are widespread in our environment, and exert an estrogenic effect on humans and other animals. Scientists are currently debating whether or not these compounds may be implicated in a worldwide increase in testicular cancer in men, and breast cancer in women. Exposure to X-rays increases risk; women who had radiation treatment to their thymus gland as children or frequent fluoroscopies because of tuberculosis or other chest problems are more susceptible. It is estimated that about 1% of the population has inherited a gene that makes the person more susceptible to cancer induction by X-ray; people who know they have a relative with the "ataxia-telangiectasia syndrome" will have a higher risk of having inherited this gene. In addition, several dietary factors have been implicated in breast cancer, such as a high content of fat or overall calories in the diet, and the use of alcohol. Recent studies have shown a possible connection between even moderate alcohol use (3 drinks a week) and breast cancer, with increased risks for heavy drinkers. See Chapters 14 and 15 for more details, including the good news that exercise and healthy eating can lower your risk of breast cancer.

Investigators have pointed out that despite the increased risk of breast cancer with estrogen use, statistics on longevity still favor the women who take postmenopausal hormones. Many more women ultimately die of heart disease than breast cancer, and hormone use gives significant protection from heart attack. On the other hand, there are many lifestyle changes we can make to reduce our risk of heart attack—quit smoking, walk daily, eat a low-fat diet high in vegetables and fruits, and take vitamins such as E, C and B complex (see Chapter 16). Breast cancer often occurs at a younger age, and there is much less we can do to prevent it. It is difficult to sort out this dilemma. I advise women with risk factors for breast cancer or serious concerns about the disease to avoid HRT, or to take it for less than 5 years. Other women should look at the self-rating scale in the next chapter of this book and make a careful assessment of their personal risks of contracting breast cancer, osteoporosis or heart disease.

All women should do breast self-exams monthly, be checked by a doctor or nurse practitioner yearly, and stop HRT if breast lumps develop, especially if they show "atypia." Mammography (X-rays of breast tissue) should be performed every year in women over 50, and every other year between 40 and 50. Having mammography regularly is important whether or not you take HRT, since it can detect very small abnormalities that cannot be felt on breast exam alone. It is best to get your mammogram from a center that is accredited by the American College of Radiology; the machine should be used only for mammograms; the technician taking the films should specialize in taking mammograms, and the amount of radiation per film taken should not exceed 300 millirads.

Breast cancer is justifiably a major worry among midlife women. It is important for all women to examine their breasts regularly and to promptly seek medical care if a breast lump is found. It is helpful to do breast exams lying down at night, or in the bathtub or shower with soap on your fingers. Put your hand behind your head on the side you are examining. Remember that most lumps are not cancer, but all should be professionally evaluated. A caffeine-free diet may decrease breast lumpiness, and a low-fat, high-fiber eating plan with lots of vegetables and soy products may reduce the risk of breast cancer. Suggestions for these changes are given in Chapter 15.

A medication known as tamoxifen (Nolvadex) is currently being tested to prevent breast cancer in women over 60 and younger women with a family history of breast cancer. Tamoxifen is a synthetic hormone that blocks the action of estrogen on the breasts. It has long been used as a treatment for breast cancer in postmenopausal women whose cancers are sensitive to estrogen. Tamoxifen's favorable side effects include possible increased bone strength in the spine and a lowered cholesterol level. Its unfavorable effects include hot flashes, an elevated rate of thrombophlebitis (blood clots in the veins), uterine cancer, and visual problems. You should not use tamoxifen to prevent breast cancer unless you are enrolled in one of the ongoing research programs.

If a breast cancer does develop, it is important to consider all your options for treatment. Consult with a surgeon or cancer specialist, and find out about new surgical techniques that remove only part of the breast if the cancer is still small. If your options are mastectomy alone or lumpectomy followed by radiation, you should give a lot of thought to your feelings about body image with only one breast, versus the short- and long-term side effects of radiation. I advise women with breast problems or breast cancer to read *Dr. Susan Love's Breast Book* for a comprehensive and compassionate discussion of breast diseases and their treatments.

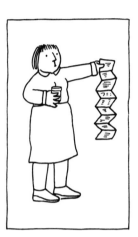

Cancer of the uterus

The main reason many women stopped using estrogen after 1975 was the finding that the medication increased the risk of developing uterine cancer. Fortunately, the cancers occurring in these women responded well to a hysterectomy and other treatments. Subsequently it has been found that the use of a progestin in the second half of each estrogen cycle allows for complete shedding of the uterine lining and very substantially reduces the risk of uterine cancer.

The cancer risk remains, however, because some doctors do not prescribe a progestin for an adequate time each month (12-14 days) and some women neglect to take it. Patients are not regularly informed about progestin use in the package insert they are given with each estrogen prescription. If you have severe side effects on your progestin pills, try natural progesterone, or ask your doctor about having a yearly endometrial aspiration to completely remove the uterine lining.

Obesity also increases the risk of uterine cancer because of the increased amount of natural estrogen formed in the body's fat cells. Menopausal women who are more than 25 or 30 pounds overweight are not advised to take estrogen until they show clear signs of lowered hormone levels, such as vaginal dryness and hot flashes. They should take a 12-day course of a progestin to promote shedding of the uterine lining which protects against this type of cancer. If bleeding occurs, some doctors suggest that they repeat the progestin every few months until there is no further bleeding.

Liver and gallbladder disease

As a rare complication, the birth-control pill induces liver tumors. It is therefore wise for doctors to check for liver enlargement in women using HRT. Women with active liver disease due to alcohol or other causes should take no unnecessary medications, including HRT.

Women taking estrogen have been found in several studies to have an increased risk of gallbladder disease. They require surgical removal of the gallbladder about twice as often as other women. Gallbladder surgery has been simplified due to new operative techniques, but it can still present risks to older women. Women most at risk for gallstones are those who are obese, have a high cholesterol dietary intake or blood level, or have diabetes, Crohn's disease, or some other rare illnesses. Native American women from the southwest frequently develop gallstones. Any woman who has these risks or knows she has gallstones should avoid HRT, and should consume foods high in fiber (whole grains, beans, and vegetables) and very low in fat.

Depression

While some postmenopausal women have found that estrogen improves their mood, others find they are depressed by it, or by the added progestin. Such depression is sometimes related to an increased need for B vitamins, and is improved by the daily use of a B-complex pill containing 25 mg of vitamin B6. If depression persists unrelated to any obvious factors in daily life, women can try switching to natural progesterone, or stopping HRT to assess differences in their moods.

Uterine fibroids

Uterine fibroids are benign overgrowths of muscular tissue which enlarge the uterus. They are stimulated to grow by estrogen. Ordinarily fibroid tumors shrink after menopause because of decreased estrogen levels and are rarely any further problem. However, HRT may cause continued growth of these tumors. Sometimes fibroids grow to a size that is uncomfortable and a hysterectomy is suggested; it is safer and easier to avoid HRT if fibroids are growing. When the uterus has shrunk to a normal size after menopause, low-dose HRT can be tried if desired.

Other potential problems

Increased rates of ovarian cancer and systemic lupus erythematosis have shown up in some, but not all, studies of postmenopausal hormone use. Both need further study before a relationship with hormones is confirmed. Ovarian cancer risk may rise after long-term use (over 10 years). Systemic lupus erythematosis is an autoimmune disease that affects women far more often than men, probably because of its relationship to estrogen. The Nurses' Health Study, in which 122,000 U.S. nurses have been followed since 1976 by investigators from Harvard Medical School, has found an increased risk of developing this rare disease among women taking postmenopausal hormones.

Increased visits to physicians

Women who take HRT generally visit their physicians more frequently for checkups. In addition to a yearly physical examination and mammogram, they should be seen if they have persistent or heavy irregular bleeding, so that a biopsy or D&C can be done to test the uterine lining. They may also need extra visits to adjust hormone doses and brands because of side effects. On the one hand, more frequent visits may result in earlier recognition of abnormalities. On the other hand, they are costly, time-consuming, and result in more medical tests, surgeries, and drugs, some of which may be harmful.

Should You Take HRT? A Self-Rating Scale 11

A fter carefully considering the pros and cons of hormone therapy, and consulting with her doctor, each woman must make a personal decision. Some will want to try estrogen because of premature menopause or sexual problems, or to alleviate hot flashes. Others may be advised by their doctors to use estrogen to prevent osteoporosis or heart disease. Some women decide that they do not want to take HRT, often because of a close family history of breast cancer or because they prefer not to take medicines. Still others may have the health problems listed below that make it unwise for them to take HRT in any case.

Women with These Problems Should Avoid HRT:
Cancer of the breast or uterus
Undiagnosed, abnormal vaginal bleeding
Blood clots in the legs or lungs at the present time
High blood pressure that is increased by HRT
Active liver disease
Gallstones or gallbladder disease

You may want to consider the following rating system to help you clarify your choice.

THE DECISION TO USE HRT: A PERSONAL RATING SCALE

This rating scale is designed to help you clarify your thinking on whether to take HRT, based on your own needs and your personal and family medical history. If you have had your ovaries removed by surgery at any age, you should give a high priority to estrogen (a progestin is not needed) because you lack the ovarian hormones that are secreted throughout life (see Chapter 3). If you are under 45 with premature menopause, you should generally take hormones until age 48 or 50; at that time you can reevaluate your use based on this scale.

How to use the scale: The advantages and disadvantages of taking HRT are listed. Each has been explained more fully earlier in the text, and is summarized in the pages which follow. Read over each summary section, and then assign a rating from 0 to +++ to each item on the scale, depending on its importance to you.

Show your rating scale findings to your doctor, so you can both determine the best course for you.

Advantages and Disadvantages of HRT—A Personal Rating Scale

Advantages

0	+	++	+++	Elimination of hot flashes and insomnia
0	+	++	+++	Elimination of vaginal soreness
0	+	++	+++	Reduced risk of broken bones
0	+	++	+++	Reduced risk of heart disease
0	+	++	+++	Possible reduced risk of colon cancer (needs further study)
0	+	++	+++	Other personal advantages _____

Disadvantages

0	+	++	+++	Possible increased risk of breast cancer
0	+	++	+++	Increased risk of uterine cancer unless adequate progestin is used
0	+	++	+++	Increased risk of gallbladder disease
0	+	++	+++	Possible growth of uterine fibroids
0	+	++	+++	Possible increased risk of ovarian cancer (needs further study)
0	+	++	+++	Possible increased risk of systemic lupus (needs further study)
0	+	++	+++	More medical visits and expenses
0	+	++	+++	Monthly bleeding or irregular bleeding
0	+	++	+++	Other personal disadvantages _____

0	=	not important
+	=	a little important
++	=	quite important
+++	=	very important

Remember to read the text before you assign the ratings.

ADVANTAGES OF HRT

Elimination of hot flashes and insomnia. As discussed in Chapter 4, the use of estrogen tablets is very effective against hot flashes and insomnia. However, these symptoms often return if estrogen is stopped.

Slow reduction of dosage can lessen but not eliminate this return. Alternative methods to deal with hot flashes are discussed in Chapter 4. Give yourself a rating of 0 to +++ depending on the importance of these problems to you.

Elimination of vaginal soreness. Estrogen is very effective in eliminating vaginal soreness due to penetration. However, minimal amounts of vaginal estrogen cream also do this, as discussed in Chapter 10. If vaginal soreness is the only symptom you want to treat, you can use very small amounts of cream twice weekly and not take estrogen pills. In this case give yourself a 0 rating. If you don't have pain with vaginal penetration, give yourself a 0 rating. On the other hand, if estrogen creams are not satisfactory and you are considering estrogen pills or the patch, rate this item with a 0 to +++ depending on its importance to you.

Reduced risk of broken bones. As discussed in Chapter 7, estrogen reduces the risk of bone fractures (osteoporosis) after midlife by about 50%. To help you decide on the importance of this problem to you, consider getting a bone-density study by DEXA or DPA, as explained in Chapter 7. This will give you a reliable idea of your current bone strength and an estimate of future fracture potential, especially if you repeat the study after a year. If bone-density exams are not available in your community, or are too expensive, look again at the table on page 66. You should know that experts in the field of osteoporosis do not currently agree on the importance of all these factors. There is much more to be learned about what causes and prevents osteoporosis in different people. Therefore, the rating you give yourself based on this table will reflect an approximate idea of your risk, not a precise one.

Check any items that apply to you on this table. If you have close women relatives with osteoporosis, or two or more checks on the Genetic or Medical Factors list, you should consider yourself at risk of developing osteoporosis. If you have no checks on the Lifestyle Factors list, your risk is lowered; but if you have one or more checks on this list your risk is increased—unless, of course, you decide to change your habits! If you are thin, especially if you are a thin smoker, your risk of osteoporosis with fractures is high. If you are dark skinned, you can consider yourself more protected from osteoporosis than light-skinned women, but you should pay attention none-theless to the factors on the table. Based on your bone-density exam or your study of this table, give yourself an overall rating for the advantage of estrogen in decreasing brittle bones. If you have made no checks on either list of the osteoporosis table, give yourself a 0 rating. If you have checked one or more risk factors, rate the importance of this item as + (a little important), ++ (quite important), or +++ (very important). This item is a difficult one. Think it over and consult with your doctor or nurse practitioner if possible. Reread Chapter 7 for more clari-fication of the issues.

Reduced risk of heart disease. The benefits of estrogen in reducing the risk of heart disease are significant. Several stud-ies show that women taking estrogen have a 50% lower risk of developing a fatal heart attack. Heart attack is the major cause of death in women over 65. If you have risk factors for heart disease, such as smoking, an elevated cholesterol level, high blood pressure, obesity, or a family history of early heart at-tack, estrogen may prolong your life. Whatever you decide about hormones, quit smoking! While estrogen may give you some protection against heart attack, it will not protect you against emphysema, or many of the cancers associated with smoking. See Chapter 17 for ideas to help you quit. Everyone can lower their risk of heart disease with daily walks and a low-fat diet. Give yourself a rating of 0 to +++ based on your personal appraisal of these factors.

Possible reduced risk of colon cancer. This benefit has shown up on several studies, and has potential importance, as colon cancer is a major cause of cancer deaths among women over 60. More studies are needed to show that the risk reduction is real, and not due to the healthier lifestyles of women taking hormones. Colon cancer risk can be reduced by a diet high in whole grains, vegetables and fruits, and low in animal fat. Regular exercise may also help in prevention. Give yourself a rating of 0 to +++ based on your personal appraisal of these factors.

Other personal advantages. Rate the importance of any other advantages of hormone therapy that you may be aware of. Some women find that it increases their sex drive, helps reduce forgetfulness, or improves their mood. Since these effects are individual, you may need to try hormones to determine their effects on you. Give yourself a 0 to +++ rating on each factor that is important to you.

DISADVANTAGES OF HRT

Possible increased risk of breast cancer. Women who take postmenopausal hormones probably have a small increased risk of breast cancer after long-term use. This risk is greater as women get older. See Chapter 10 for more details. Other risk factors include a close family history of breast cancer, not having borne children, a late first birth, being tall, a high-fat diet and the use of alcohol. Women with a prior breast biopsy showing "atypical proliferation" are also at greater risk. Give yourself a rating of 0 to +++ based on your personal appraisal of these factors.

Increased risk of uterine cancer unless an adequate progestin is used. Women with a uterus who take estrogen without an added progestin (10 or more days per month) are at increased risk of uterine cancer. This risk persists for some years after estrogen is stopped. Vaginal ultrasound and a yearly endometrial biopsy may be protective, but are not fully studied as yet. See Chapter 10 for more details. Give yourself a rating of 0 to +++ based on your personal appraisal of these factors.

Increased risk of gallbladder disease. Gallstones, gallbladder pain, and the necessity for surgical removal of the gallbladder have occurred with greater frequency with estrogen use in several studies. Women most at risk for gallstones are those who are obese, have high cholesterol levels in the blood, or have diabetes, Crohn's disease, or some other rare illnesses.

Native American women from the southwest frequently develop gallstones. A high-fiber diet protects against gallbladder disease. Give yourself a rating of 0 to +++ based on your appraisal of your risks.

Possible growth of uterine fibroids. Estrogen can cause uterine fibroid tumors to grow larger. While these benign tumors usually shrink after menopause, they can remain large or continue to grow when HRT is taken. If you do not have fibroids, you can give this item a 0 rating. If you have them, discuss this question with your health care provider, and give yourself a rating between + and +++.

Possible increased risk of ovarian cancer. Increased rates of ovarian cancer after 10 years of use have shown up in some, but not all, studies of postmenopausal hormone use. This needs further study before a relationship with hormones is confirmed. A family history of ovarian cancer may also increase your risk; childbearing, breast feeding and prior birth-control pill use lower your risk. Give yourself a rating of 0 to +++ based on your personal appraisal of this possible risk.

Possible increased risk of systemic lupus. Systemic lupus erythematosis is an autoimmune disease that affects women far more often than men, probably because of its relationship to estrogen. The Nurses' Health Study, in which 122,000 U.S. nurses have been followed since 1976 by investigators from Harvard Medical School, has found an increased risk of developing this rare disease among women taking postmenopausal hormones. Further studies are needed to confirm this finding. Give yourself a rating of 0 to +++ based on your personal appraisal of this possible risk.

More medical visits and expenses. Women who use postmenopausal hormones need checkups every 12 months, and at other times if complications occur. They will probably have more laboratory tests, and will spend money every month buying medications. Give yourself a rating of 0 to +++ based on your feelings about this.

Monthly bleeding or irregular bleeding. When estrogen is taken after menopause, with a progestin added for 12-14 days per month, a monthly flow usually continues, necessitating the use of pads or tampons. This flow rarely causes serious cramps. When estrogen and a progestin are taken together every day, there may be irregular bleeding for up to 6 months, but after this most women experience very little bleeding at all. Give yourself a rating from 0 to +++ depending on your feelings about this. Women with premature or early menopause may welcome monthly bleeding, and put this item in the advantage column.

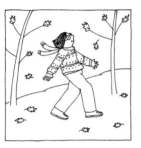

Other personal disadvantages. Rate the importance to you of any other disadvantage of estrogen therapy that applies to you. Some women find it difficult to remember to take daily pills, do not like the way they feel on HRT, or think that such use of hormones is against nature's plan for their bodies. Rate your personal appraisal of these disadvantages from 0 to +++.

When you have rated each item on the table of Advantages and Disadvantages of HRT, look at the table for some time and think about it. You need not compare your total score for advantages and disadvantages. The table is not designed to give you a numerical score, but to summarize the data and let you judge how strongly you feel about the benefits and risks of HRT as they are currently known.

Be sure to discuss your questions and conclusions with your doctor or nurse practitioner, both now and as your knowledge increases and your feelings change. Remember that many women have tried hormones and then stopped them; others have decided to use hormones years after menopause. Your decision does not have to be final. Remember also the alternative treatments for menopausal problems discussed in this book.

PART II

POSTMENOPAUSAL ZEST (PMZ)...
HOW TO FIND IT AND KEEP IT

*I'm not exactly sure what lies ahead for me ... this new
young woman. It's a brand new role for me. All this freedom
to be myself at long last. To really be myself. Not what
someone said I should be ... not what someone expected me
to be. I don't know what is around the bend ... but I do
know that I'm on the path that takes me there ... my feet are
willing and light ... my spirit is free ... and I am
feeling ... wonderful.*

—Gloria, age 50, after her menopause

As menstrual periods stop, women enter a time in their
lives which can be vital and new. Margaret Mead, the
well-known anthropologist with an interest in women's roles,
coined the term "postmenopausal zest" for this period.

What is this state? Zest is a quality that gives our lives
relish, stimulation, and keen enjoyment. How do we find and
keep a sense of zest for living in midlife? Everyone knows
some older people who have it—who are vital and involved in
the world around them. We also know people of the same age
who are depressed, ailing, or reclusive. In this section we will
consider ways to find and keep a zestful outlook in the second
half of life. Some of these concepts have been touched on
earlier in this book in relation to special problems of menopause, but most ways to keep zestful are as useful to men as to
women.

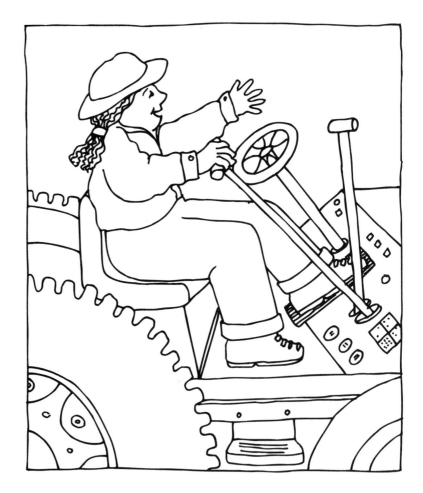

Beliefs about Aging: Unfolding and Growing, or Dying on the Vine?

12

The greatest discovery of any generation is that human beings can alter their lives by altering their attitudes of mind.

—*Albert Schweitzer*

Aging is the term for a continuous process of growth through life.

—*Maggie Kuhn*

*J*anet was very involved in running her farm, and at 55 she was attending extension courses at night to learn more about new methods of organic farming. Her husband had died of a sudden heart attack when she was 48. Both her daughters had gone to the state capital to work. At first she was overwhelmed and thought of selling the farm, but gradually she began to see that she could handle it herself with some new techniques, different cash crops, and the help of a young couple who came to live with her. She realized that she came from a long line of strong farm women who had overcome great hardships in coming to this country and living off the land. She enjoyed the challenges of outdoor work and farm management, and found she could do many things she previously left to her husband. When people admired her work she was fond of saying, "These past years have sure taught this old dog some new tricks."

Rebecca lost her job as a secretary after 20 years when the firm went bankrupt. She was 52, and lived alone. She managed to find occasional

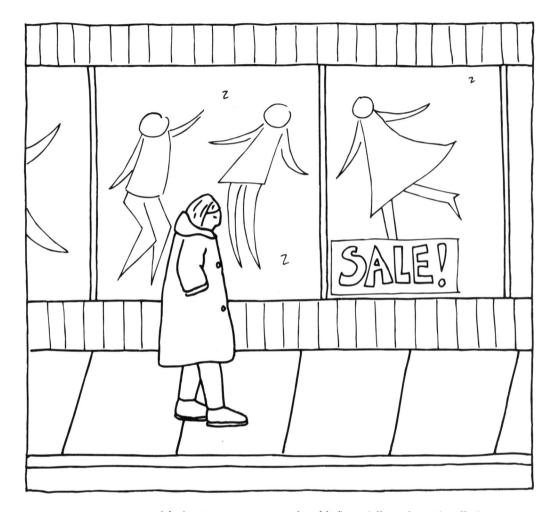

jobs in a temporary agency but felt financially and emotionally insecure. She called her son on the phone daily and wanted to move in with him, but he had a wife and small child and did not welcome the idea, although he did send her some money every month. Rebecca increased her daily dose of estrogen and took antidepressants, but she still felt terrible. She saw no future for herself. She felt she had alienated most of her old friends by refusing to go out with them or crying so easily. At the mental health clinic they suggested she be hospitalized and consider shock treatments, but she had no insurance and was frightened by this idea. Rebecca remained depressed, often contemplating suicide but being restrained by her religious beliefs and her attachment to her son and grandchild. After a few years, she slowly began to improve. A friend gave her some back copies of Prevention *magazine, and she started taking vitamins and eating healthier food. She felt a little better, but still had trouble seeing herself as valuable or important in any way. Besides her son and her part-time jobs, she had very few connections to the world around her. She didn't see how she could possibly start any new activities or get any new interests at this stage in her life.*

We are subtly but profoundly influenced by the beliefs our culture holds about aging. Often our view of other women or ourselves in the menopausal years is a composite of how we saw our own mothers and other family members, and what we absorb from the media. Many women have negative memories of their own mothers' menopausal symptoms, and a strong dread of aging. Others have positive, powerful, or serene role models in their families.

It is worth spending some time understanding what your own inner views of menopause and aging may be. Close your eyes and picture a woman of 50, in her menopausal years. What does she look like, how does she feel, how does she move and speak? Write down three adjectives to describe this woman. Do the same for a woman of 60, and then one of 70. Visualize them in your imagination, and then describe each with three adjectives. Look over what you have written, and get an idea of your own fantasies and beliefs about aging. Do you like these women? Do you want to be like them as you age? If not, what do you want to be like when you are 50, 60, and 70?

Play the game again, and visualize yourself at each of those ages. Write down three adjectives to describe yourself at 50, 60, and 70 the way you really want to be. Now look at your two lists. Is your second list—with your personal ideals— different from your first list? What this exercise can do is show you that you don't have to be like your imaginary pictures of an older woman if you don't want to be. You can be your unique self, growing older in your own fashion.

Although our culture may have a stereotyped view of men and women at various ages, projected in television, movies, and advertisements, real people are incredibly diverse. We are usually happier if we value our uniqueness and do not try to make ourselves over to fit the cultural mold. Women who do not accept the prevalent belief that their worth as females depends on youthful sex appeal can value wisdom and strength in middle age. However, if you listen to messages like, "You can't teach an old dog new tricks"—you can't learn a new skill, sport, language, or instrument after age 15 or 25 or some other cutoff date—you will make these prophecies come true for yourself.

To break away from the negative belief systems, it helps to find friends who are excited about life after 50 and talk to them about their outlooks, activities, and plans. Find out about organizations like the Gray Panthers, composed of people of all ages who want to change society and combat ageism. Find the nearest chapter of the Older Women's League (OWL), or Elderhostel, which promotes educational adventures for older adults at academic institutions worldwide. Gradually you will see a more positive view of human potential in aging which you can incorporate into your consciousness. Let your fantasy and imagination dwell on these new role models instead of negative stereotypes. Think of Representative Pat Schroeder, the Honorable Barbara Jordan, former Surgeon General Joycelyn Elders, and authors Betty Friedan or Gloria Steinem. These women are some of my role models—you will want to find your own!

STAY CONNECTED TO THE WORLD AROUND YOU

Numerous studies of aging have shown that people connected to a network of others are happier and live longer. While spending time alone is important for quiet self-renewal and creativity, it can be a problem for depressed people who spend it watching television or drinking. Connections to the natural world are also important—animals, plants, walks in the park, and hikes in nature. These activities keep us aware of the web of life and help to combat depression.

Community and political involvement are important tasks for the second half of life. We need to use our experience to

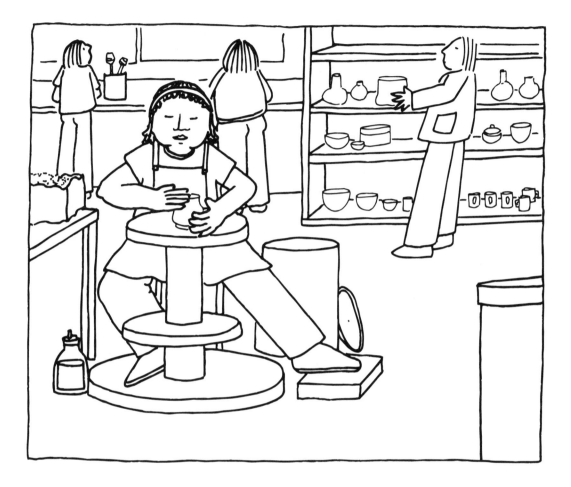

help direct the larger society in which we live, in whatever way seems most appropriate. Voting is important, but many people can give more than a vote to a cause or organization they believe in. Such individual efforts are the lifeblood of our democratic society, and can give great meaning to those who participate in them.

Middle-aged people who believe in their abilities to keep on learning and giving are doing many things in our society. They are returning to college, sometimes finishing a degree at 60 or 70 that they couldn't pursue in their 20s. They are involved in community affairs, politics, or crafts, in addition to holding down jobs. Sometimes they are finding new ways to earn income from their interests. Women who have been mothers, in particular, must redefine themselves in midlife when the parent role has ended. This is important as a bridge to the future, to keep life vital into old age.

Think about the "shouting out" sessions mentioned in Chapter 8. One of our important life jobs is to keep discovering and growing until we die. As one sage woman puts it, we must uncover our inner design. This means discovering who we are—amid or beyond our many roles as worker, parent, spouse, or lover—and what really gives our lives meaning. What excites us and makes us grow? What can we best give to the world around us? Such answers are obvious to some people but hard for others to find. Answers vary at different times in our lives. Getting even a partial answer to these questions is energizing. Knowing where you are going in life is an important part of postmenopausal zest.

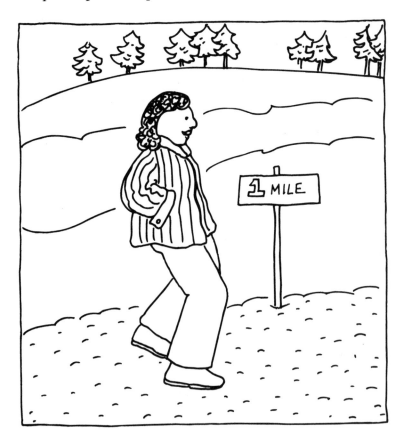

Relaxation: Calming Down and Letting Go 13

The softest thing in the universe
Overcomes the hardest thing in the universe.
That without substance can enter where there is no room.
Hence I know the value of non-action.
Teaching without words and work without doing
Are understood by very few.

—Lao Tsu

Life is constantly challenging, both physically and psychologically—and cannot be otherwise. Our innate urges to survive, relate to others, learn, and master our environment cause change and conflict. The idea that life can be lived without stress, or that happiness is found in perpetual relaxation is a common misinterpretation of the aims of stress-reduction techniques. It has been aptly named "The Elysian Fields fallacy."

What we need is the ability to alternate between being alert and energetic on the one hand, and relaxed and calm on the other. This sounds obvious, but many people have difficulty letting go of the tension they accumulate during the day. They are perpetually switched "on" and can only turn themselves "off" with alcohol, tranquilizers, or exhaustion and fitful sleep. Some of the reasons for this are obvious. Urban living is

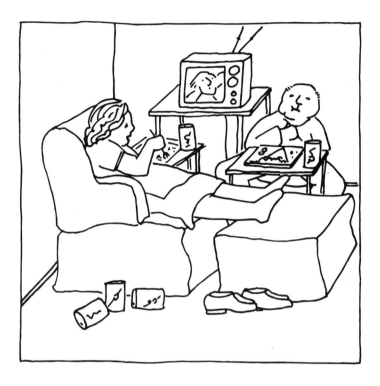

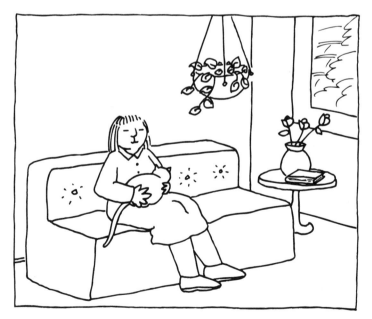

crowded, noisy, mechanized, and rushed. The media bombard people with sounds of urgency and scenes of violence or disaster. Competition and "hurry sickness" are an important part of our culture. "Hurry sickness" is a term discussed by Drs. Friedman and Rosenman in their book, *Type A Behavior and Your Heart;* it refers to pervasive feelings of urgency and time pressure which may contribute to heart disease and other common illnesses of contemporary life.

It is overly simplistic to say that heart disease, cancer, allergies, or ulcers are "caused" by excessive stress alone. There are many other genetic, environmental, and lifestyle factors

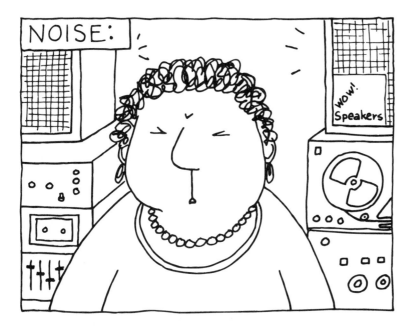

involved in these illnesses. However, we can say that many illnesses are aggravated by prolonged, excessive tension—whether it stems from noise, rush, and overwork, or from fear, anger, and self-blame. Conversely, sick people often recover faster, with less pain and disability, when they learn to get rid of excessive tension. Animal research shows that stress or fear depress the immune system, making the body more vulnerable to infectious agents or cancer.

Let's consider some of the factors in everyday life which can be changed to lower tension and restore balance to our nervous systems.

Noise is an obvious place to start. Many people are constantly bombarded by noise, which causes tension, fatigue, and blood pressure elevation. Noise at work and in cities may be unavoidable, but noise at home can be minimized. Anyone who feels overstressed should experiment with turning off the television, radio, and loud music, and living with silence. Even short periods of silence during the day are helpful to enable our nervous systems to rebalance. In Quaker tradition, silence is used for worship, and for the beginning and end of business meetings and ceremonies. It enables the participants to renew themselves, hear their inner spirits, and go forth to be effective in dealing with the problems of the world.

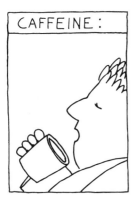

Many people repeatedly drink coffee, tea, or colas during the day, giving themselves a caffeine high that comes from stimulation of the adrenal glands and the central nervous system. It is more difficult to relax under the influence of a stimulant drug. When people cut down on caffeine consumption or eliminate it completely, the results are striking. They frequently feel less stressed. They learn to identify when they are really tired and need to rest or relax. Moreover, they can relax more easily without needing a drink.

Both caffeine and alcohol can be pleasurable and useful drugs, but they are both physically addictive. We can be energized or relaxed without them and experience a quicker return to a natural state of being.

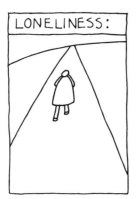

Loneliness and social isolation can be stressful. While many people need to spend time alone in order to relax or get in touch with their inner resources, most people need and enjoy a network of supportive friends and family. Working too hard, being too competitive, or moving too frequently makes it hard to maintain a circle of close friends. Recent research indicates that people with close-knit ties to family, friends, or religious or other social groups have lower mortality rates from all diseases than people who are socially isolated. It has been postulated in this regard that one reason women live longer than men may be related to their greater interest in social and family ties. Men and women who have the personality pattern that has been connected with heart attacks—competitive, hurried, impatient, and striving—may be more vulnerable because they cannot make good connections with other people.

Overwork is another common cause of excess tension. It is clear that hard work is necessary for survival, especially in times of economic difficulty. Change and technological progress make it hard to keep up in any field without constant efforts to learn new things and alter our belief systems. However, each person must assess whether she or he is taking on so much that constant feelings of rushing or incompleteness result. If there is literally no time in your day to relax, eat an unhurried meal, or talk with friends, your life plan may need reassessment. Quakers consider it important to limit one's work life to have enough time for family, friends, and activities connected to the Meeting. One well-known cancer specialist insists that his patients spend an hour a day doing something that involves play and fun. Norman Cousins advocated "laugh therapy." It's better not to wait until you're seriously ill to follow these prescriptions!

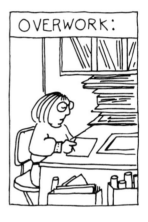

Inner tensions can be as destructive as those generated by the outside world. Anxiety, fear, grief, anger, self-blame, and poor self-image are words describing complex and unpleasant feelings that assault us and cause distress. Counseling with a trained psychotherapist is often an effective approach to these problems. In addition, many people have found the consistent use of relaxation techniques very helpful.

RELAXATION TECHNIQUES

The goal of relaxation techniques is to enable people to return to a calm center after periods of activity. We understand intuitively that noise, conflict, anxiety, and hard work activate a part of our nervous system that is prepared for action in the struggle for survival. Another part of our nervous system functions when we feel peaceful, quietly aware, receptive, and relaxed. This part enables us to digest our food, sleep soundly, enjoy sexuality, and obtain relief from muscular pain. Pulse rate and blood pressure decrease. The immune system works more efficiently to prevent or overcome disease when we are relaxed. Many creative thoughts and important insights occur during times of quiet.

Relaxation exercises help in two ways: first, to return to a state of calm after episodes of anger, fear, or intense action, instead of feeling residues of emotional turmoil all day; and second, to maintain inner balance most of the time, even dur-

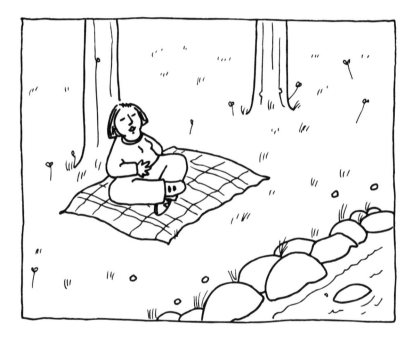

ing great stress, by having a sure sense of one's center and meaning. This comes with time, practice, and self-knowledge.

Many methods of relaxation are helpful; different ones are suitable for various needs and people. Meditation, silent prayer, yoga breathing methods, massage, biofeedback, using a relaxation tape or lying quietly in a warm bath are all ways to relax. Herbert Benson describes a simple breathing technique in his popular book, *The Relaxation Response*. A professor of medicine at Harvard University, Benson distilled the essence of meditation techniques from many cultures and religions into his prescription. Basically, it is this: Sit quietly and comfortably with your spine straight and your eyes closed. Silently say the word "one" in your mind with every exhalation. Focus your mind on your breathing and the word "one." When other thoughts come to you, let go of them. Develop a receptive and passive attitude. Do this for 10 minutes, twice a day. As you turn off the outside world with its noise and pressures, and turn away from your own thought processes, your body will enter a state of relaxation that has remarkable restorative effects.

I highly recommend *The Relaxation Response*. A perceptive reviewer said this book "can show those of us who are trapped in the Twentieth Century how to lower our blood pressures, change our harassed personalities, and, perhaps, even save our lives." To this I can add that many problems of middle age, including fear of aging and low self-esteem, are also helped by the relaxation response. People with certain illnesses, such as cancer, may want to use a relaxation technique that specifically relates to their problems. In this case, relaxation is combined with positive images of self-healing.

In addition, readers with life-threatening illness may be interested in the book *Choices in Healing—Integrating the best of conventional and complementary approaches to cancer*, by Michael Lerner. This book contains an overview and analysis of many forms of treatment—medical, nutritional, psychological and spiritual—written by a scholar who has surveyed the field with compassion and objectivity. The names and addresses of conventional and complementary healing centers throughout the U.S. are included.

Carolyn, age 49, was a nonstop talker and a successful businesswoman. She came to my office because of abdominal pain, digestive problems, and fatigue. She drank a lot of black coffee to keep her going at work, and smoked cigarettes to keep from overeating. She had written out a long list of physical symptoms that were troubling her, from headaches through back pain to cold feet. Almost none of her natural body functions were working smoothly. After listening to her problems and conducting a physical examination, I suggested that we try a brief relaxation exercise as a model for what she could do at home. Carolyn found it very difficult to keep her eyes closed and not to talk for 5 minutes. "I couldn't wait to stop so I could tell you about another problem I have," she said. Then she laughed at herself and added, "I guess that's a part of my problem, isn't it?" Carolyn reluctantly embarked on some changes in the way she lived, including a 20-minute tub bath before dinner with the telephone unplugged, every night. In the year to follow she tried several relaxation techniques, and found that biofeedback worked best for her because she could measure her progress on the machine. She ultimately bought an inexpensive biofeedback machine to use at home. Most of her physical problems were resolved without drugs, and she slowly cut down on her coffee and cigarette use. She learned to be silent without feeling anxious, which made it easier for her to get along with other people.

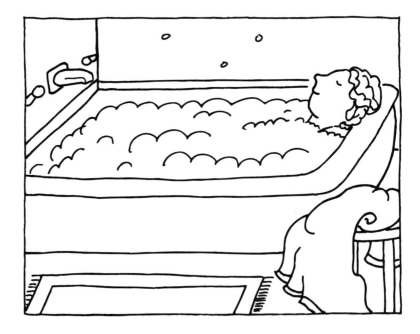

Use It or Lose It: Exercise in Midlife 14

There is no drug in current or prospective use that holds as much promise for sustained health as a lifetime program of physical exercise.

—Dr. Walter Bortz,
Professor of Medicine, Stanford University

Our bodies are magnificently designed to move. But after a lifetime of sitting—in schools, offices, cars, and homes—we often end up pain-ridden and diseased. Doctors are slowly coming to understand that many of the changes we have attributed to aging are simply those that accompany physical inactivity. When young people stay in bed, they experience the same degenerative changes in heart and lungs, bones, muscles, body fat content, and digestive and nervous systems that we usually associate with growing old.

When middle-aged people exercise they can prevent, retard, or reverse many of these changes. The benefits of exercise include a reduced risk of heart disease, osteoporosis and possibly breast cancer, easier weight control, improved appearance, decreased pain from many conditions, less depression, and better sleep. Let's examine these factors individually.

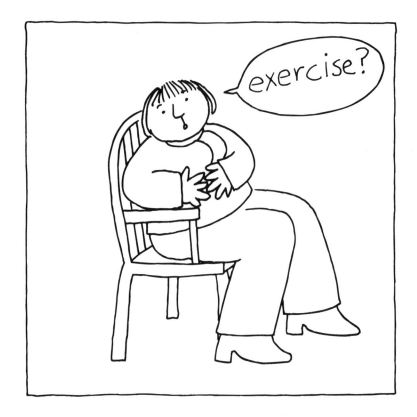

HEART DISEASE

Exercise helps prevent heart attacks. Though heart attack is the leading cause of death among women over 65, it is not inevitable. The kind of heart disease we have seen in this century is relatively new—arteries blocked by deposits of waxy cholesterol have never before been seen with such frequency. Our overconsumption of rich animal food, smoking, and physical inactivity seem to be the culprits. In past centuries, heart disease was mainly due to rheumatic fever and other infectious diseases, or birth defects, many of which can now be prevented or surgically remedied. Yet the only lasting hope for the new heart disease—cholesterol-plugged blood vessels—is lifestyle change. Surgery to clean out or replace the blood vessels to the heart muscle carries a surgical risk and only buys time. The vessels can become blocked again if the patient doesn't cut down on fat and start to exercise.

The combination of a low-fat, high-fiber diet and regular exercise has a remarkable effect on the heart. Exercise makes the heart a more efficient pump, causing more blood circulation with each contraction and sending more oxygen to the muscles. As a result, you can do more without getting tired. This is what aerobic exercise is about. Any exercise is aerobic if it helps to condition the heart, lungs, and muscles to work more efficiently, or allows you to consume more oxygen during activity, and thereby experience less fatigue. If you start a brisk walking program, for example, you may feel tired after 1 mile at first. But a month of brisk walking conditions you so you can walk 4 or 5 miles with ease. Your heart will have been trained to become a better pump. It will beat more slowly when you are resting, because it will be stronger and send out more blood with each beat. It will have developed new blood vessels within the heart muscle to nourish itself with oxygen. Your chances of developing serious heart disease will have decreased. Equally important for the here and now, you will have developed more endurance and feel less fatigue throughout your daily activities. When you run for a bus, carry groceries upstairs, or folk dance, you will feel strong and capable rather than exhausted.

If you have exercised all your life, by all means continue daily during menopause and beyond. If you have been fairly sedentary in the last month or two, begin with a walking program. Work up to 30 minutes a day of brisk, uninterrupted walking in comfortable, flat, walking shoes. Walking is an excellent form of aerobic exercise which you can continue for life with great benefit. So is swimming, or riding a stationary bicycle—a good alternative for stormy weather. As you start out with this program, check with a physician to assess the health of your heart and blood vessels. This is especially important if you have any history of heart disease, diabetes, high blood pressure, or chest pain. A doctor's checkup is very important for middle-aged people who have been inactive and plan to start jogging, aerobic dance, or competitive sports. It is

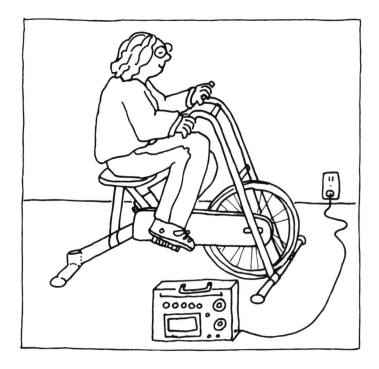

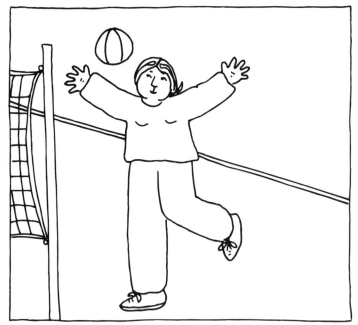

safer to begin with a walking program and gradually get conditioned.

Readers interested in a full discussion of the benefits of exercise to the heart will enjoy the books of Kenneth Cooper, the cardiologist who started the worldwide enthusiasm for jogging. In *The Aerobics Way*, Cooper gives detailed charts for working up to optimal exercise times for each age group and each type of activity. For people ages 50 to 59, Dr. Cooper recommends working up to walking 2½ miles in 37 minutes, 4 times per week, or riding a stationary bicycle 25 minutes, 4 times per week, with the controls (resistance) set so that a pulse rate of 150 is reached. Cooper's basic premise is that the heart becomes a more efficient muscular pump if you keep it trained. Just as our arm and leg muscles get stronger as we use them and weaker if we rest them, so does our heart muscle. A strong heart is a comforting companion in the second half of life.

The good news about movement is that anything you do is better than doing nothing. Your heart will benefit even if your exercise is spread out in short segments throughout the day. People with desk jobs should wear walking shoes to and from work and walk some of the way whenever possible. Do some walking during your lunch break, and use the stairs instead of the elevator for a few stories. Disabled people can often find a form of activity, such as swimming or water exercise, that will stimulate their hearts. Swimming, bicycling, walking, gardening, housecleaning, dancing and many leisure activities all count. If you play golf, stay out of the little electric carts!

But what about the waxy deposits of cholesterol in the blood vessels nourishing the heart? How does exercise prevent clogging these vessels? In a couple of ways: it encourages the formation of a larger network of blood vessels to nourish the heart muscle. In addition, it makes the blood less likely to clot by increasing natural anticlotting factors. Conversely, inactivity makes clotting more likely. This is another reason why heart attacks and strokes are less likely if you regularly exercise.

OSTEOPOROSIS

The brittle bone problem of middle-aged and elderly women is helped by exercise. Recent studies show encouraging results in preventing and reversing osteoporosis when women take up a consistent exercise program. The subject of osteoporosis is thoroughly discussed in Chapter 7, and will be only briefly reviewed here. Bone fractures and back pain from compressed vertebra are both outgrowths of progressive loss of calcium from the bones, which occurs in women after menopause. Black women appear to be more resistant to this condition, perhaps because of their stronger bone structures. Latina women from Central America also have fewer fractures. About

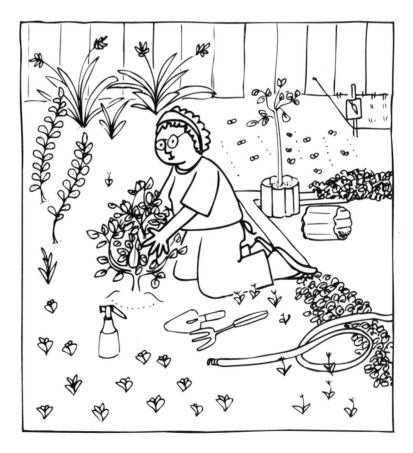

25% of White and a smaller proportion of Asian women develop painful fractures from slight injury after menopause. The most effective approach to osteoporosis is prevention, and exercise is a key factor. People who are inactive, or confined to their beds, quickly lose calcium from their bones. Conversely, people who vigorously use their limbs and muscles develop thicker, stronger bones.

Middle-aged and elderly women need a daily walking program for their lower bodies. A recent study from Tufts University showed that women past menopause who consistently walk a mile or more daily have slower bone loss in the legs and all over their bodies than sedentary women. Since energetic walkers can cover a mile in 15 to 20 minutes, you can see that this is not a time-consuming suggestion.

Men and women lose muscle strength with aging, and need to combat this loss with exercise. Whatever builds muscle will build bone. Research indicates that muscle-strengthening exercises for the back, abdomen, shoulders and arms are important measures to prevent spinal osteoporosis. A racket sport, energetic gardening, swimming, modified pushups, drumming or lifting weights may be what you would enjoy. Strength training for people over 70 is considered the best way to prolong independence, and is now being used in progressive nursing homes. Exercise trainers say that working with free weights, such as dumbbells, is more effective for the whole skeleton than using exercise machines that isolate specific muscle groups. It is important to start slowly, and have some expert advice as you begin a strengthening program. You can do weight training at home if you go to a sporting goods store and buy a set of 3- and 5-pound dumbbells (later you may want to add heavier weights). The book *Getting in Shape* (see *Suggestions for Further Reading*) has practical advice on strength training for women and men, as well as stretching and walking. Follow the directions, turn on some music, and begin! It is important to lift 2 or 3 times a week to make gains, and to wait 1 to 2 days between strengthening workouts. Brisk walking is a good activity for the days off, so that you alternate between cardiovascular fitness and body strengthening.

Even sick people and hospitalized patients should move around. Bones begin to rapidly lose calcium with bed rest. Enlightened doctors prescribe leg exercises to their postoperative patients and encourage them to start walking soon. If you spend the day at home ill, remember to move as well as to

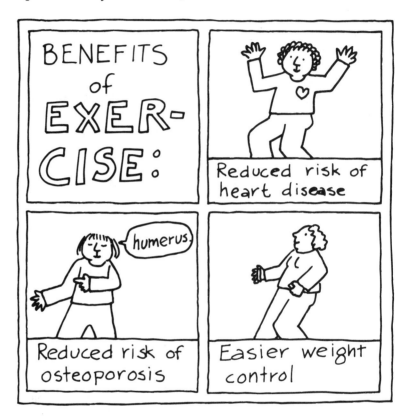

sleep. Get up every few hours, stretch, walk, and work your muscles gently. Your recovery will be easier, and your bones will stay strong.

CANCER PREVENTION

Intriguing new studies have linked lifetime exercise habits with lower rates of breast cancer in women and possibly with prostate cancer in men. For men, the benefits of regular exercise may have to do with lower testosterone levels and therefore less stimulation of the prostate gland. For women, studies indicate that strenuous exercise throughout life results in fewer monthly cycles in which ovulation takes place. This may play a role in the lower rates of breast cancer that occur among athletes. The message here is to encourage your daughters to be physically active, and to continue your own exercise program throughout life. If you begin to exercise in your 30s or 40s you may get less of a protective effect against breast cancer, but the benefits for your heart and bones will still be significant.

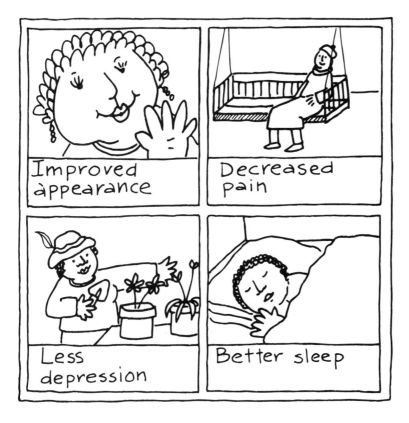

WEIGHT CONTROL

It's difficult to keep your weight in balance if you don't exercise. The small amount of food needed to sustain you in an inactive state keeps you chronically hungry and often undernourished. When small animals are kept in cages without an exercise wheel and given unlimited food, they tend to become obese. If they are given the opportunity to exercise along with unlimited food, they usually balance their intake with their energy output and maintain a normal weight. We function the same way. Weight loss is far easier if the dieter follows a daily program of walking, swimming, dance, or other movement.

In and after menopause, women should not be too thin. The obsession with being slender in our society leads to great problems in self-image for most women at most ages. In the second half of life it is especially counterproductive, because thin women have less estrogen and greater problems with hot flashes, vaginal soreness, and osteoporosis (see Chapters 4, 5, and 7). This is not to say that real obesity is helpful; it has definite health risks also. Find the middle way for yourself—a weight that feels good and can be maintained.

APPEARANCE

The person who works out with vigorous movement and stretching keeps a look of vitality and suppleness in the second half of life. A stiff body is not an inevitable part of aging. When middle-aged people start to exercise, amazing changes in their appearance are noticeable very quickly; a new grace comes from flexibility and energy. Yoga, dance, and Tai Chi are especially good forms of movement to impart youthful balance and grace throughout life.

DEPRESSION, MOODS, AND SLEEP

Exercise has subtle but extremely beneficial effects on our moods. The physical, muscular activity of vigorous movement stimulates the brain, causing the release of substances which produce euphoria or "high" good feelings. Depression and physical pain are lessened. This is one reason why many joggers, dancers, or walkers get addicted to their activity. Some psychotherapists prescribe aerobic activity for depression and even go jogging with their patients. Any of us can experience a "natural high" through movement. Many people find they are able to give up tranquilizers or antidepressant drugs when they begin daily exercise. They sleep more soundly at night, even in the menopausal years when sleep is often troubled by hot flashes. Anyone with insomnia should try daily exercise as one form of treatment.

Stretching exercises also help to counteract emotional problems. Tension is always accompanied by physical muscular contraction. Chronically contracted muscles are tight and often sore. As we learn to stretch and relax our muscles, our minds become calmer. The amazing benefits of hatha yoga are related to this principle.

HOW TO START EXERCISING

The public has been exposed to lots of information about the benefits of exercise, and clearly it has made an impact. Joggers and bikers are all around us. Most adults, however, still lead fairly sedentary lives in our society, except for occasional weekend flings. The two most important realizations about exercise are these: First, you have to find activities you really enjoy or you won't keep them up; and second, you have to plan exercise into every day—just as you plan meals, shopping, and going to work. If you don't consciously make time for exercise you probably won't get it, especially if you live in a city.

Energetic Activity
>   vigorous walking, hiking
>
>   jogging, race walking
>
>   dance, jazzercise, aerobics
>
>   bicycling
>
>   stationary bicycling
>
>   jumping rope
>
>   swimming
>
>   racket sports
>
>   energetic gardening or farm work
>
>   sawing or splitting wood manually
>
>   cross-country skiing
>
>   weight lifting or working out in a gym

Stretching
>   dance
>
>   yoga
>
>   many floor exercises

Finding an exercise activity that you really enjoy takes some introspection. Consider whether you want to take a class and be with people at a set time, or be by yourself at your own schedule. Do you want to exercise inside or out, with music or without it? Do you enjoy team sports and competition, or do you want individual exercise with your own thoughts and your own agenda? Was there anything you did in childhood that would really be fun to take up again, like swimming, jumping rope, biking, or dancing? Do you need different things on different days? Do you want to join a gym and work out on your lunch hour or after work, then have a sauna? Do you want to ride a stationary bike or use a rowing machine while you watch the news? Go over the table of energetic exercise and stretching, and think about those that seem right for you.

Women with disabilities that prevent the usual forms of exercise can often find interesting substitutes. Confer with a physical therapist for the best ideas to suit your condition.

Swimming and water aerobics are sometimes possible. You may be able to work out with an arm bicycle (a wheel turned by your arms against graduated resistance, usually found in physical therapy centers); this gives aerobic benefits to the heart as well as upper body strength.

Remember to start slowly with any exercise if you have been inactive; patience and persistence really pay off. Above all, look at exercise as a way to put fun into your day, because the right kind for you will do just that.

Charlene was very unhappy about her body. At 53 she considered herself 40 pounds overweight, and she saw that she was gaining more each year. Yet she ate rather sparingly compared to many of her thinner friends, which seemed very unfair. Every piece of cheese turned to fat on Charlene! She longed to go swimming at the community center pool, but felt much too embarrassed to show herself in a bathing suit. A friend urged her to join an exercise class, but for that she would have to wear a leotard! Even walking had gotten uncomfortable because of her weight. One day a belly dance teacher came to the community center to do a show. She was almost as fat as Charlene, but incredibly supple and sexual. Amazingly, she seemed happy with her body. Charlene thought about the dancer a great deal. She called a local studio that taught belly dancing and discussed it anonymously on the phone. The woman told her that belly dancers were proud of their bellies and that she should come try out a class. She bought a tape and practiced daily at home or in class. Gradually she began to feel at home in her body again, for the first time in years. She became graceful and supple, and even lost a few inches and pounds. Many of her physical discomforts went away. Above all, she started to carry herself with pride.

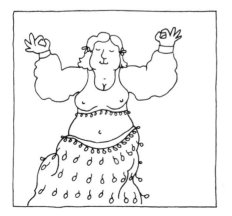

Nutrition: All about Eating and Drinking

15

You are what you eat.

—Anon.

*And when you crush an apple with your teeth, say to it in
    your heart*
"Your seeds shall live in my body,
And the buds of your tomorrow shall blossom in my heart,
And your fragrance shall be my breath,
And together we shall rejoice through all the seasons."

—Kahlil Gibran

Eating the right food is an extremely important part of
staying healthy and feeling connected to the natural world.
New information about substances in plant foods known as
phytochemicals, which give protection against many cancers,
heart attack, osteoporosis and other diseases, make this chapter one of the most important in this book. Read on for an
explanation of why our grandmothers, or great-grandmoth-
ers, were right when they made meals with a lot of different
vegetables and fruits from the back garden or the green grocer
down the street.

The optimum diet for menopause and middle age is high
in vegetables, whole grains, fruit, and foods high in calcium.
Such a diet can supply plenty of nutrients without causing
obesity or heart disease. One advantage of this healthy diet is

that it is delicious; another is that it is less expensive than a diet centered around meat and packaged or prepared foods. Above all, a plant-based diet is extremely healthy. When people change to a better diet, they often notice that many problems slowly disappear. Energy increases, weight stabilizes, hair gains luster and stops falling out, skin looks better, gums stop bleeding, and constipation disappears. Let's look at the individual elements of a healthy diet and understand their pros and cons. At the end of this chapter are some recipes and suggested menus.

FOODS

Whole grains

Grains are delicious and can be cooked in many ways: whole—as in brown rice; cracked or rolled—as in oatmeal; or ground into whole-grain flours. The grain family includes wheat, rye, triticale, rice, oats, barley, corn, millet, buckwheat (kasha), quinoa and wild rice. Although grains have been a staple food for most of recorded human history, they have mistakenly acquired the reputation of being high in calories. Perhaps this is because of what we put on them: butter, cheese, gravy, and

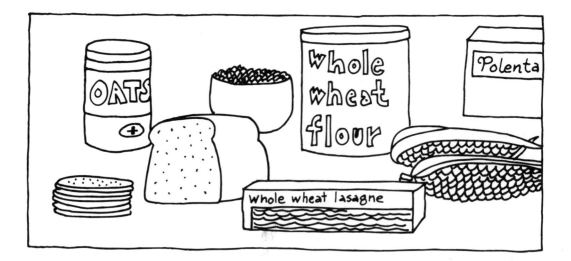

mayonnaise! A slice of whole-grain bread has about 90 calories, a cup of cooked brown rice about 200 calories. Asian people, who live on a rice-based diet, are mainly slim, in contrast to westerners on a meat(fat)-based diet. The fiber in whole grains helps you eat more slowly and fill up naturally, so you won't overeat. In general, it is the fat in our food that makes us fat, not the grains, potatoes, and vegetables.

The medical advantages of whole grains are worth thinking about. Everyone is aware that something called fiber is good for you and relieves constipation. Fiber, the indigestible part of plant foods, is found in different forms in grains, beans, vegetables, and fruits. People who eat a diet high in fiber have a lower risk of contracting cancer of the colon, and also have fewer problems with many gastrointestinal diseases, such as diverticulitis, hiatus hernia, and appendicitis. They also have lower cholesterol levels in the blood, even after eating the same amount of cholesterol in their food. This decreases their risk of heart attack.

It is also possible that a high-fiber, low-fat diet protects women against breast cancer. Women in Asia and Africa consume much less fat and three times more fiber than we do, and have a lower incidence of breast cancer than American women. Vegetarian women in the United States, whose diet is lower in fat and higher in fiber, have less breast cancer than meat-eaters. Many people add bran to their food in order to get more fiber. This is a good first step, but eating 100% whole grains makes more sense for your health. Bran is only one of the elements removed in making white flour or white rice. The germ of the wheat or rice kernel is the other part removed; it contains the B vitamins, vitamin E, and other nutrients.

Here are some guidelines for using whole grains: Buy or make your own whole-grain bread without added white flour or sugars. Use brown rice, rolled oats (not the instant kind), rye crackers, fresh corn, corn tortillas, polenta, and buckwheat groats (kasha). Start the day with a whole-grain cereal. Use whole-wheat pasta, available at health food stores or food co-ops. Read a book like *The New Laurel's Kitchen* for easy ways to cook with these grains. Gradually shift away from white bread, cakes, donuts, and pastries to these healthier foods. If you like

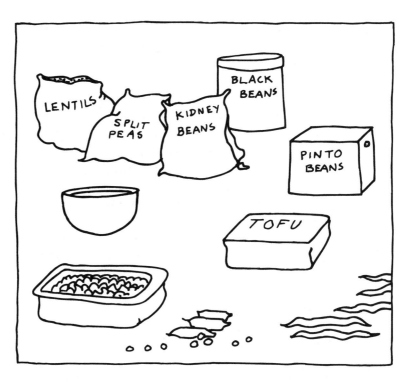

to bake desserts, use whole-wheat pastry flour, which is entirely interchangeable with the white variety. Try plain popcorn for a snack.

Beans

Beans are excellent foods for several reasons. They are high in protein and low in fat. Any bean combined with any grain gives you protein of the same quality as meat, fish, eggs, or milk. For example, a serving of baked beans or split pea soup combined with rice, bread, or corn gives you protein as complete as that in meat. Vegetarians are well aware of this, and often find they can easily maintain their desired weight.

Another advantage of beans is their high fiber content. The fibrous cover around the bean slows its breakdown in the digestive process, so its nutrients are absorbed more slowly than other foods. Beans are considered the ideal food for people with diabetes because their slow, regular absorption minimizes the need for insulin. If you are bothered by intestinal gas when you eat beans, cover the dry beans with plenty of water and let them soak for 12 hours. Throw away the soaking water, rinse the beans, and cook them in fresh water. This process eliminates certain starches that cause intestinal gas. Also, try fresh or frozen beans and peas, bean sprouts, and soybean foods like tofu and tempeh (found in oriental markets and natural food stores).

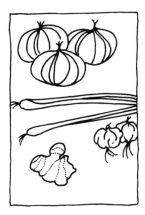

People who get much of their protein from beans and grains are helping the world food supply as well as their own health. Sixteen pounds of grain and soybeans must be fed to beef cattle to produce one pound of meat. If more of us ate the grain and beans instead of the meat, huge amounts of agricultural land in this world could be planted with basic crops for the hungry. This idea is developed in John Robbins' impressive books, *Diet for a New America* and *May All Be Fed*; it has caused many people to examine their usual ways of eating.

Soybeans

It has long been known that soybeans provide a complete source of protein, containing all the essential amino acids that we need in the proper amounts. This is one reason why they have been an esteemed human food for thousands of years in Asian cultures. Soybeans also deserve special mention because they have a key role in the most exciting new discovery in nutrition—the finding that many substances in plant foods help to prevent cancer, heart attacks and other diseases. These newly discovered substances have been called *phytochemicals*, which simply mean plant chemicals; they are not proteins, carbohydrates, fats, or vitamins, but they seem to have great health benefits.

In recent years scientists have found that unique phytochemicals, found only in soybeans, have the ability to block the growth of certain cancers, and also to give substantial protection against heart disease and osteoporosis. These substances, known as *isoflavones*, have a chemical structure similar to estrogen. Although isoflavones are much weaker than estrogen, they can both mimic and block some of the activities of estrogen in the human body.

Isoflavones are believed to protect against cancer in several ways. Because they act as a weak estrogen, they may attach to estrogen receptors in the human breast and block the stimulating action of a woman's own hormones. In addition, young American women given soy protein on a daily basis have been found to have a longer menstrual cycle—for example, they would go for 30-31 days instead of 28 days from the beginning of one period to the next. Over a reproductive lifetime, this could result in substantially fewer days of exposure to the high estrogen levels of ovulation. Isoflavones inhibit the growth of many kinds of cancers by blocking the development of new blood vessels around a malignancy, and thus preventing nutrients from reaching the cancer. Scientists studying these compounds feel that the frequent use of soy products, such as green vegetable soybeans, tofu, miso, and soymilk may explain the much lower rate of breast and prostate cancer and lower proportion of deaths from these diseases in China, Japan and Korea.

Soy foods also give some protection against osteoporosis; the extent of this protection is still being studied. Soy protein causes less calcium loss in the urine than animal protein, and the isoflavones in soy may have a directly beneficial effect on bone. A medication known as *ipriflavone* is a synthetic version of soy isoflavone; ipriflavone has been found to prevent post-menopausal bone loss and is currently being evaluated in Italy and other European countries.

Protection against heart disease by soy foods is another exciting new finding. Soy has the ability to lower total cholesterol and LDL cholesterol, the culprit in causing blockages in the arteries. A recent Italian study looked at the effect of soy protein in children with a familial disease characterized by very high cholesterol levels. A low-fat diet alone was of little help, but the addition of soy protein (instead of animal protein) was able to reduce their cholesterol levels by 26% in a month. These data have aroused intense interest among nutrition researchers.

An excellent book for the general public on these new discoveries is *The Simple Soybean and Your Health,* by Mark and

Virginia Messina. The Messinas have a wide breadth of knowledge on the biochemistry and uses of soybeans—their book clearly explains the current scientific research on the soybean and gives recipes for including soy foods in your daily diet. If you want to keep up with ongoing research, you can also subscribe to a newsletter called *The Soy Connection,* 10525 N.W. Ambassador Dr., Suite 202, Kansas City, MO 64153. Dr. Messina writes a column in this newsletter.

Many people want to know how much soy they should eat to get its benefits. I recommend that all Americans eat some soy foods in their daily diets—for example: a serving (2-3 ounces) of tofu or tempeh 3 times a week, and on alternate days a blender drink of soymilk and banana, or soynuts as a snack. You can also use a small amount of miso paste instead of salt to flavor your dishes. Tempeh is an Indonesian meat substitute made from soybeans, and miso is a Japanese condiment made of fermented soybeans—both are available in natural food stores.

Vegetables
Vegetables have always been pushed by nutritionists and mothers because of their abundance of vitamins and minerals. Now we are also learning that they have an abundance of different phytochemicals that may protect against cancer, infections,

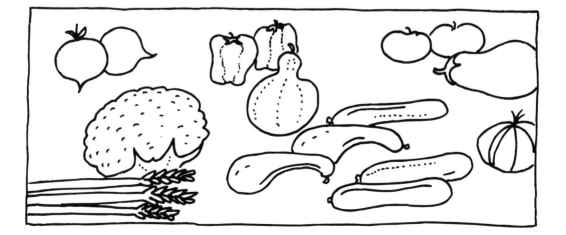

heart attacks, and stroke. In our long evolutionary history we relied a great deal on the gathering of tubers, leaves, grains, beans, berries, seeds and nuts for survival. We probably have inbuilt mechanisms that make us dependent on the plant foods we gathered in abundance for many thousands of years. It is tragic that so many of us have turned away from these foods to fill up on burgers, fries, soft drinks, chips, candy and ice cream. These new foods give us more than enough calories for growth, but not enough phytochemicals to keep us in optimal health.

In the course of our daily digestion and metabolism, our bodies use oxygen and generate molecules known as *free radicals*—which can change genes and possibly cause cancer in the long run. Our bodies also have enzymes which deactivate free radicals, but deeply colored vegetables, soybeans and many fruits contain so-called *antioxidant* substances which help this process along. People with high intakes of vegetables and fruits are getting abundant antioxidants such as vitamin C, beta carotene and other so-called carotenoids; hundreds of carotenoids have been found in plants, many of which have important biochemical functions in our bodies. There are many studies indicating that people who eat the most fruits and vegetables have substantially lower cancer rates than those who eat the least. Antioxidants in vegetables also have been shown to protect against heart disease. Caretenoids found in deep-green, leafy vegetables, such as spinach, kale, collard and mustard greens, also protect against a common form of visual loss in older adults, known as *macular degeneration*, and other antioxidants protect against cataracts. The coming years will probably bring considerable new information about foods that are protective against a variety of diseases.

There is evidence that vegetables in the cabbage family— broccoli, Brussels sprouts, cabbage, cauliflower, kale, and col- lards—protect against cancer because of the presence of a substance known as *sulforaphane*—which triggers the body's production of enzymes that detoxify cancer-causing com- pounds. Broccoli seems to be the most potent vegetable in this family.

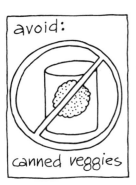
avoid:

canned veggies

Citrus fruits, berries, grapes, apples, garlic, onions, leeks and chives, whole grains, green leafy vegetables of all kinds, yams and winter squashes, tomatoes, peppers—the list of plants with potential cancer fighters is fairly comprehensive. The phytochemicals in each food are different, so you must eat a varied diet to get the maximum benefits.

Garlic and onions can lower levels of serum cholesterol and decrease the tendency of the blood to clot. Similar effects against clotting are seen with ginger root and certain mushrooms.

Vegetables can be eaten raw in salads or lightly steamed. Water in which vegetables have been cooked should be kept and used as broth, because it is high in vitamins, minerals and the newly found nutrients discussed above. Don't throw away your cooking water!

Sprouting is another way to obtain delicious food high in nutrients. As sprouts grow, their vitamin content increases, providing the benefits of fresh vegetables even in winter in northern areas. Anyone can make bean sprouts in the kitchen, from lentils, aduki beans, mung beans or many seeds. No other fresh crop is so easily obtained. Cover ¼ cup of small beans like lentils with water and soak in a glass jar for 12 to 24 hours. Rinse the beans and invert the jar after covering its mouth with cheesecloth or a fine-meshed screen. Keep the jar inverted on your dish-drying rack, rinsing the beans twice daily. The sprouts will be visible in a few days; eat them raw in salads or throw them into pasta or stir-fried vegetables at the end of cooking, so they stay crisp.

Potatoes and sweet potatoes are excellent foods which should not be avoided because of their alleged tendency to cause weight gain. They are not the problem—it is the oil, butter, and sour cream with which they are often prepared. Potatoes are best steamed or baked, and can be served with yogurt and chives or other seasonings. They are good sources of protein, vitamin C, and potassium, an important mineral for people with high blood pressure.

Sea vegetables are not used in western cooking but are high in necessary trace minerals. You can buy small amounts of dried and flaked kelp, dulse and other sea vegetables at a natural food or oriental grocery store. Add a small amount to rice, salads, soup or stews. Books on Japanese, Philippine, or Hawaiian cooking give more details on the use of sea vegetables.

As much as possible, avoid canned or pickled vegetables, as their salt content is unusually high. Frozen vegetables are a better alternative when fresh produce is not available. Don't forget to make your own bean sprouts in the winter!

Fruits

Fruits are an excellent source of vitamins, minerals, beneficial phytochemicals and pleasure. Many can lower your risk of cancer, heart disease, intestinal problems and high blood pressure. Eat fruit for snacks and desserts, instead of donuts, ice cream, or pastry. When your friends and co-workers bring out cake, Valentine candy, or other sugary snacks, you can open a desk drawer, purse, or refrigerator and produce a tangerine or some dried figs. Most of us find it is important to be supplied with healthy "reward" foods if we are to turn down the "treats" that lead to tooth decay and obesity.

It's true that fruits have a high sugar content, along with their vitamins and minerals. But their fiber content slows down the eating process and makes us full faster. In addition, the

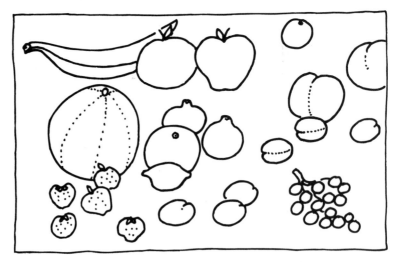

fiber of raw fruits has a stabilizing effect on blood-sugar levels. If you eat 2 whole apples, your blood sugar will rise, just as it will if you drink the juice of those apples without their fibrous pulp. Two hours after the whole apple snack your blood sugar will be back to normal. However, 2 hours after the apple juice, your blood sugar will be significantly lower. This is because more insulin was released from your pancreas to help digest the quickly absorbed apple juice. The body responds to the juice alone in the same way it responds to simple sugar in soft drinks or desserts. The downswing of blood sugar after the initial rise makes many people feel relatively shaky, and hungry soon again. The lesson here is—enjoy the whole fruit. Don't make a regular habit of drinking fruit juices.

Most of us wonder how to avoid the pesticides sprayed on produce. Wash fruits and vegetables carefully before eating them. When possible, find a farmer's market where you can get locally grown produce, and look for stores that sell unsprayed or organic products. These markets and farmers deserve our support. One advantage of local produce is it has more nutrients because it is picked riper and only briefly stored. And finally, if you have a backyard or space for pots, start growing a few vegetables and fruits at home. The connection to the earth and the good eating are both nourishing.

Meat, poultry, and fish

All are tasty additions to a healthy diet in middle age, but none should be center stage. To have a low fat content in the diet, and thereby to decrease the risk of heart disease and cancers of the colon, ovary and breast, we should use meat as a flavoring for grains and vegetables rather than as the centerpiece of the meal. Oriental cooks do this by cutting up meat or fish and stir-frying it with onions, garlic, and vegetables. There are many other ways of changing to a low-fat, low-meat diet, such as making vegetable stews, casseroles, or soups using lean meat as a flavoring.

When cutting down on meat, it is not necessary to compensate with eggs and cheese; in fact, this defeats the purpose of achieving a lower fat content in the diet. Remember that a

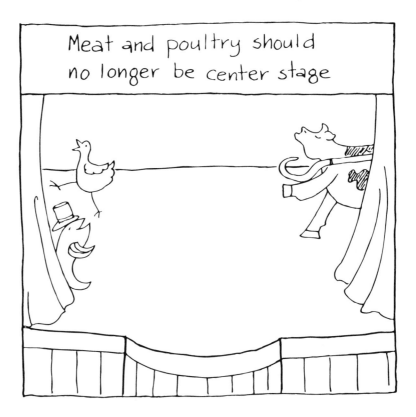

bean and whole-grain combination, or soybeans alone, provide high-quality protein without added fat. You can eliminate
meat entirely and be healthy! Vegetarians have good health
records, with lower rates of heart disease and cancer than
meat-eaters.

If you do like meat, how much is enough, and what kinds
are best? Many heart specialists agree that middle-aged people
should not eat more than ¼ pound of lean meat daily. Trim all
visible fat from red meat and choose the leanest cuts. Discard
the skin of poultry. Don't use gravy. Avoid bacon, ham, lunch
meat, and pressed or processed meats—they are high in fat,
salt, and chemicals.

Frying or broiling meat at a high temperature develops
certain cancer-causing products. Use a lower temperature for a

longer time, or cover the meat and let it stew in its juices, staying at the boiling point.

Another reason to minimize flesh foods in midlife is that they may contribute to osteoporosis, or brittle bones (see Chapter 7). There is evidence that high-protein diets cause a loss of calcium from the body. Several studies have shown that vegetarians have less osteoporosis than nonvegetarians. To prevent osteoporosis, it is better to get most of your animal protein from low-fat milk products. You can eliminate milk, eggs, and all animal protein from your diet and still be very healthy in your adult years. Complete vegetarians, known as *vegans*, get their calcium from broccoli, kale, collards and other plant foods (see table on p. 176), and all the protein they need in beans and whole grains. A supplement containing vitamin B12 is usually a good idea, as discussed in Chapter 16.

Fish is the one flesh food that has a protective effect against heart disease, by virtue of the special kind of fat it contains. The oil in fish has been shown to lower blood levels of cholesterol and to counteract the tendency of blood to clot. Nutritionists often suggest that middle-aged men and women include fish in their diets once a week, emphasizing the fatter fishes like salmon, mackerel, trout, and herring. If you eat canned fish, read the label carefully and drain any vegetable oil that is sometimes added. The midlife woman interested in health could consider getting all her animal protein from fish and low-fat milk products instead of meat and poultry. Alternatively, she can become a vegetarian. Both ways are helpful.

The beneficial fat found in fish, known as *omega-3 fatty acid*, or alpha-linolenic acid, is found in only a few plant foods. One accessible source is flax seed, which can be bought in natural food stores. Grind the seeds in a coffee or spice grinder and eat 1 or 2 tablespoons daily if you don't eat fish—you can sprinkle ground flax seed on cereal, salads or cooked vegetable dishes. Some people find that skin problems and painful joints are improved by adding more omega-3 fatty acids to their diets.

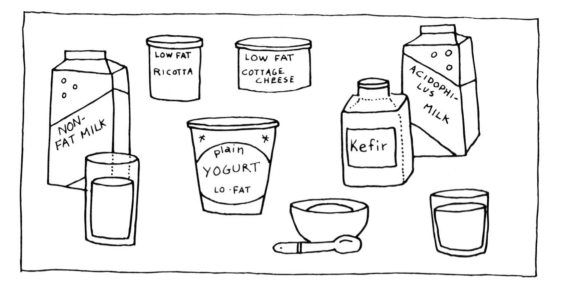

Common Foods High in Calcium

Food	Amount	Calcium Content
skim-milk powder	¼ cup	400 mg
1% fat milk	1 cup	350 mg
calcium-fortified soy milk	1 cup	300 mg
low-fat yogurt	1 cup	300 mg
low-fat cottage cheese	1 cup	120 mg
collard greens, cooked	1 cup	360 mg
sardines, canned	8 medium	350 mg
blackstrap molasses	2 tablespoons	280 mg
sesame seed meal (tahini)	¼ cup	270 mg
kale, cooked	1 cup	200 mg
salmon, canned with bones	3 ounces	170 mg
broccoli, cooked	1 stalk	160 mg
tofu (soybean curd)	4 ounces	150 mg
corn tortillas	2	120 mg
calcium-fortified orange juice	1 cup	320 mg

When making soup stock from bones, add 1 or 2 tablespoons of vinegar during the boiling process. The acid in the vinegar will dissolve the calcium out of the bones, providing a soup stock unusually rich in calcium.

Milk, yogurt, and cheese

Nonfat and low-fat milk products are helpful for midlife women because of their calcium content. However, some adults lack the ability to digest milk sugar (lactose), and experience cramping, gas, and diarrhea after drinking milk. Sometimes such people can eat small servings of cultured milk such as yogurt, buttermilk, acidophilus milk, and kefir, where the milk sugar is partially digested already by the fermenting bacteria. Lact-Aid, a product sold in pharmacies, also predigests milk sugar and does so without making the milk sour. Soy milk can be used as a milk substitute; I advise the new, light soy milk (1% fat, which means that 18% of its calories come from fat) for drinking, cereal and for cooking.

Adults (and children over age 2) should avoid most high-fat milk products such as butter, sour cream, ice cream, whipped cream, half-and-half, and large amounts of whole milk. About 75% of the calories in hard cheeses of all kinds are fat; hard cheeses should be used in small amounts for flavor. Low-fat cottage cheese (uncreamed), low-fat and nonfat yogurt, and nonfat milk are good choices, useful in cooking as well.

Many cultures do not use milk products and some westerners avoid them because of digestive problems, arthritis, or a dislike of factory farming. Since calcium intake is so important in midlife women, those who avoid milk should eat plenty of the other high-calcium foods listed in the table every day. Aim towards eating about 300 mg of calcium at each meal from the foods listed in this or other nutrient tables. *The New Laurel's Kitchen* (Ten Speed Press, 1986) is an excellent vegetarian cookbook with useful tables of the calcium content in most foods. Be sure to read the next chapter's discussion of calcium supplements as well.

Eggs

Eggs are a high-protein food many people enjoy and they are very useful in cooking. Because of the high cholesterol content of egg yolk, eggs have become controversial in recent years. Most cardiologists endorse the concept of a prudent diet where egg yolks are used in moderation—say 3 or 4 per week in

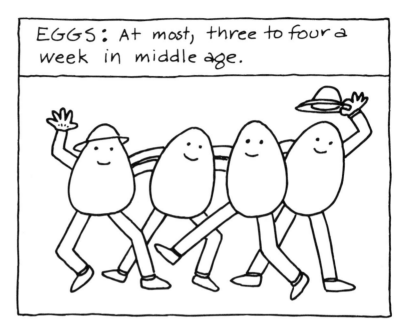

EGGS: At most, three to four a week in middle age.

middle age. Yolks should be completely avoided by people with an elevated cholesterol or any problems involving blocked arteries in the heart, the brain or the legs. It is much healthier to eat eggs poached, boiled, or baked in food than fried in fat. Cheese omelets or soufflés are very high in fat and cholesterol and should generally be avoided. Powdered or dried eggs in various packaged foods should be avoided, as there is evidence that processed, dried cholesterol may do more damage to blood vessels than the cholesterol in fresh food.

People who are limiting their fat and cholesterol intake often use egg whites and completely avoid yolks. Farmers who raise their own chickens and eat their own eggs should know that chickens fed only grains and plant foods have about 50% less cholesterol in their eggs than chickens fed meat meal, fish meal, and poultry by-products.

FAT, SUGAR, AND SALT

Fats

Butter, margarine, oil, mayonnaise, cream, and lard are very high in calories, yet low in essential nutrients. Typical Americans consume about 40% of their calories in fat. This pattern of eating has been strongly linked to heart disease, stroke, and various cancers, especially cancer of the breast, ovary and colon. Since these diseases account for more than half the deaths in the United States, it is important for our society to change their eating patterns, moving toward a much lower fat diet. Individuals can do this without major disruption if they do it thoughtfully.

For health, we do not need to add any fat or oil to our foods. Enough fat is obtained from whole grains, vegetables, a few nuts and seeds, and lean or low-fat animal products to satisfy our needs and allow us to absorb fat-soluble vitamins. Most people, however, want to have some fat in their diets for taste and a feeling of being full. Therefore, the key concept is to use fat sparingly. Use just a little butter, peanut butter, or cheese on your sandwich, with lots of vegetables and sprouts. Try eating bread or potatoes with a little olive oil and garlic rather than butter or margarine. Use just a little oil in frying and avoid deep-fried foods. (You can sauté food in broth or water instead of oil.) Make salad dressings with more lemon, vinegar, spices, and low-fat yogurt, and less oil or mayonnaise. Cut down by a third or more on the fat (butter, oil, egg yolk, and so on) required in recipes, and buy a low-fat cookbook.

The public has been confused in recent years by recommendations on which oils are the most healthful. Many people know that animal fats such as butter and lard, and certain vegetable fats (coconut and palm oils) are high in saturated fat; they thereby tend to raise cholesterol levels and promote heart disease. Polyunsaturated oils such as safflower or corn oils were once in favor, because these oils will lower cholesterol levels. However, while diets high in polyunsaturated oils lower heart-attack risk, they may raise the risk of cancer, as shown in some human and animal studies. Olive and canola oils, known as *monounsaturated oils*, are currently preferred, because they seem to lower the risk of heart attack without increasing cancers. Olive oil consumption was linked with lower breast cancer rates in a study from Greece. However, you should not use large amounts of monounsaturated oils either—they do contain some saturated fats and are loaded with calories. It is wise to use only small amounts of fat in any form.

Margarines have less saturated fat than butter, but they are no better for your health. Vegetable oils are "hydrogenated" to form margarine; this process of adding hydrogen atoms to the oil thickens it and creates a type of fat that is unnatural for the body, has an unfavorable effect on cholesterol, and has been linked to heart disease. Partially hydrogenated vegetable oils are found in many store-bought candies, cakes, pastries, cookies, crackers, and potato chips as well as in leading brands of peanut butter. I suggest you carefully read labels and avoid foods with hydrogenated oils. Palm oil, palm kernel oil, and coconut oil should also be avoided.

Eat seeds and nuts sparingly—they can be healthy but have a high fat content. Walnuts and almonds, without added

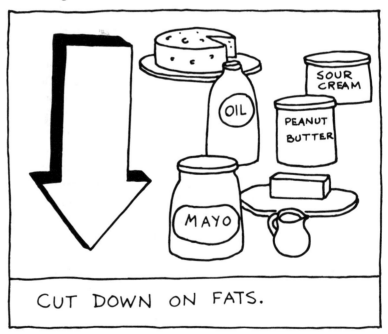

CUT DOWN ON FATS.

salt or oil, have been found to lower cholesterol levels; sun-flower seeds and pumpkin seeds add richness to vegetable dishes; think of these as a treat rather than a staple food. Be very cautious with coconut or avocado. Fill up on whole grains, vegetables, and fruits.

Ice cream is a major problem in terms of fat! This all-American dessert and snack was never a nutritional star, but in recent years has been worsened by the addition of many additives, fillers and chemicals. I suggest avoiding it completely, getting it out of the freezer, and having fat-free frozen yogurt or fruit sorbet as an occasional treat.

People who consciously change to a low-fat diet notice several pleasant differences. Many remark that they feel lighter, more energetic, and less sleepy after meals. They spend more time eating, and eat a greater volume of food, since low-fat foods are usually high in fiber and require more chewing. Yet they lose weight more easily and often stabilize at a weight considerably lower than before, without consciously dieting. Low-fat foods fill you up with fewer calories.

Dieters, take note! Fat contains 9 calories per gram, whereas carbohydrates and protein contain 4 calories per gram. When you eat carbohydrates, such as potatoes, rice, pasta, bread, vegetables and fruits, most of these foods are transformed into body heat and a compound known as *glycogen*. Glycogen is stored in your muscles and liver, and serves as a reservoir of energy throughout the day. The fat you eat is mainly stored as fat in the body. Carbohydrates do not have the same power to make you gain weight as the very concentrated sources of calories in fat. The good news from this is that you can lose weight without going hungry, by avoiding fat and eating lots of healthy carbohydrates as well as some low-fat protein foods such as beans, fish, skim milk or light soy milk. Losing weight need not make you feel constantly hungry, shaky, or weak.

It's difficult, but not impossible, to find low-fat foods when you eat out. Much restaurant food is rich in butter, oil, cheese, and sauces. The conscientious eater can look for health-food restaurants and Asian restaurants, steamed or broiled fish without added butter, salad or baked potatoes with dressing on the side, and similar simple dishes. When

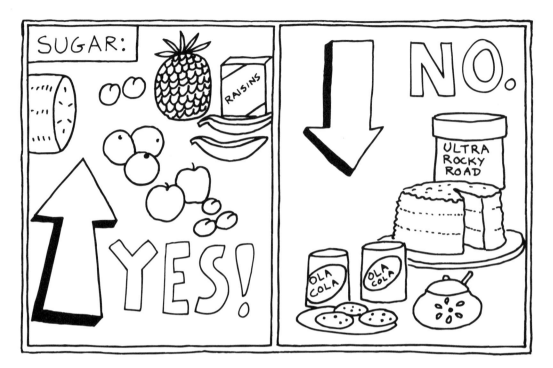

making air-travel reservations, ask for a vegetarian or low-cholesterol meal, or fresh fruit salad. Take some whole-grain crackers and fruit in your handbag.

The recommendation to change to a low-fat diet is extremely important for staying well in the second half of life. It requires self-education and vigilance, but it's very rewarding in terms of one's energy and resistance to disease. It would be best to begin a low-fat diet in childhood, but middle age is not too late! The risk of heart disease increases after menopause, and a low-fat diet (plus exercise) is more important than ever.

Sugar

Simple white sucrose and its variations such as fructose are added to cakes, cookies, soft drinks, ice cream, candy, cold cereals, and many other packaged foods. Honey, maple sugar, and molasses are added to many health-food products. All these foods promote tooth decay and tooth loss, and represent substantial calories without nutrients. According to recent estimates, the average American eats 128 pounds of sugar per year! Sugar and syrups account for about one-fifth of our total calorie intake. When 40% of our calories come from fat and 20% from sugars, it's easy to see why many people in our society are overweight and prone to chronic illness.

For optimum health, eat sugary foods very sparingly, and satisfy sweet cravings with fresh and dried fruits. Many people do this by clearing all sugary foods out of their kitchen—from cookies to ice cream and soft drinks. They find they cannot avoid eating these foods if they are in the house. If you crave sweets, stock your kitchen with fruit, including prunes, raisins, dried figs, and dates. Take some to work, and reward yourself for saying "no" to morning donuts. The sugar you get in fruit is supplemented by vitamins, abundant potassium, and other minerals which aid in its digestion and in many body processes. Fruit has fiber but no added fat or salt. People who eat fruit but avoid refined sugar have far less tooth decay and other diseases of civilization.

Many people feel really addicted to sweet foods, in the sense that they crave ice cream, cookies, or chocolate daily and feel deprived without them. Usually these foods were associated with love and good times in childhood, and the association is hard to sever. It is best to work on this gradually, cutting down on sugary foods rather than cutting them out. Meanwhile, explore the beauty and bounty of whole, natural foods and the exotic world of fruits. Focus your mind on the positive qualities of what you are gaining, not on what you are giving up.

Many people trying to lose weight use sugar substitutes such as aspartame and saccharin in desserts, soft drinks, and coffee. Saccharin is controversial because it causes bladder cancer in experimental animals. While this effect has not conclusively been shown in humans, the FDA requires a warning label about cancer on products with saccharin. Attempts to ban saccharin in the U.S. have been countered by great public pressure for its continued availability. Aspartame is a more recent sugar substitute which appears in diet soft drinks, packets for coffee and tea, and many diet desserts. A number of neurologic side effects have been reported by people who habitually use aspartame in soft drinks and diet foods—

dizziness, headache, insomnia, anxiety, depression, panic attacks, and even seizures. If you eat artificial sweeteners, look carefully for side effects. Better still, satisfy your sweet tooth with an orange or a date.

In general, chemicals in food should be avoided. We already take in a considerable number of chemical substances from pesticides, herbicides, preservatives, and additives in food. It stands to reason that we should limit our intake of any chemical we don't need, especially if it is suspected of having adverse effects. In addition to avoiding artificial sweeteners, we should avoid artificial flavoring, coloring, and most other additives. Become a label reader and don't eat chemicals unless you know they are safe. The Center for Science in the Public Interest (CSPI, Suite 300, 1875 Connecticut Ave., N.W., Washington, DC 20009-5728) puts out an excellent newsletter (*Nutrition Action Healthletter*) that explains the possible risks of food additives, and gives an entertaining overview of nutrition and food policy.

People who want a low-calorie alternative to diet soft drinks can drink low-sodium mineral water mixed with a little fruit juice or a squeeze of lemon. Delicious, low-salt vegetable juices are also available. With enough consumer demand, such healthful alternatives may soon be found in vending machines.

Salt

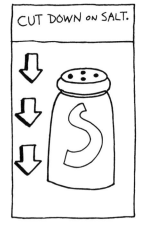

The sodium in table salt (sodium chloride) and many packaged foods can contribute to high blood pressure and osteoporosis. Recent research has shown that the chloride part of sodium chloride may also raise blood pressure. For optimum health, most people should limit salt intake, and instead flavor food with onions, garlic, lemon juice, herbs, and spices. The body does require sodium, but usually we get enough of this element in vegetables, fruits, grains, and animal foods. In societies where little or no salt is added to food, there is virtually no problem with high blood pressure. Conversely, in societies like Japan, where food is highly salted, high blood pressure and stroke (a complication of high blood pressure) are very common.

From the perspective of good health, most food in the United States is oversalted. Not everyone develops severe blood-pressure problems, but certain groups are more susceptible to it. Genetics plays a part here—people with family histories of high blood pressure are more likely to develop the problem if they salt their food. African-Americans seem to be especially at risk for high blood pressure—possibly due to genetic susceptibility to salt intake.

Limiting salt means cooking with little or no added salt and using herbs and other flavorings instead. It means avoiding much processed food, like canned soup, canned vegetables, pickles, olives, salted nuts, potato and tortilla chips, soy sauce, tamari, miso, and many packaged foods including packaged desserts. Any hard cheese should be used sparingly, because it is high in sodium as well as fat. Restaurant food is often overloaded with salt, although many cooks will prepare low-salt and low-fat dishes if asked.

Salt is an acquired taste. Children brought up without it grow into adults who don't crave it, and adults can gradually condition themselves to enjoy food with less added salt. People who have curtailed their salt intake are amazed at how salty ordinary American food tastes to them.

The drug treatment of high blood pressure often has undesirable side effects, such as fatigue, dizziness, or decreased sexual drive. There may also be unexpected, long-term side effects to the powerful drugs now being used to combat hypertension. Though these drugs are necessary for some people, the medical profession is currently reevaluating their use. Many people can successfully bring down blood pressure without drugs by lowering their salt and fat intake, losing weight, drinking very little alcohol, eating a diet high in vegetables, fruits, and calcium, exercising, and using relaxation techniques like yoga, meditation, and biofeedback.

Because of their high potassium content, fruits and vegetables are important in a program to reduce blood pressure. Potassium is an element similar to sodium, essential to life, but having the opposite effects on hypertension. Diets high in potassium and low in sodium tend to bring blood pressure down. Potassium is abundant in winter squashes, beans of all kinds, potatoes, leafy greens, and many fruits. When steaming or boiling vegetables, use the cooking water later as broth in order to retain all the potassium and other nutrients.

Packaged foods now have labels which include the amount of sodium per serving, to help you evaluate your daily intake. Most people should not use more than 2,400 mg daily. Note that many canned or dried soups contain 800 mg or more per serving, and frozen dinners often have 1,000 mg or more.

ALCOHOL AND CAFFEINE

Alcohol
Alcohol can produce pleasure, relaxation, sleep, relief from pain—and disease and death as well. The effects depend on the amount used and the metabolism and personality of the user. The menopausal woman, and middle-aged people in general, should treat it as a recreational drug to be used with care and respect. Our bodies cannot take as much abuse when we are 50 as when we were 20—hangovers last longer and feel worse! Let's examine the positive and negative effects of alcohol so we can make good decisions.

The positive aspects of alcohol for many people are that drinking enhances sociability, brings relaxation, and tastes and feels good. In addition, there is evidence that small amounts of alcohol increase a type of blood fat called HDL (high density lipoprotein) which protects against heart attack. A report from the Nurse's Health Study in the United States showed that middle-aged women consuming 3 to 9 drinks a week were 40% less likely to develop heart disease than nondrinkers. A drink is defined as 5 ounces of wine, 12 ounces of beer, or 1 ounce of hard liquor. Women who drink moderately have slightly higher estrogen levels in their blood, and thereby gain some protection against osteoporosis. Studies of people who live to age 90 or 100 have shown that many of them drink alcohol, usually in a social context with family and friends.

Positive remarks about alcohol must always be balanced with a recognition that this drug has also brought terrible personal tragedy and social disruption to our society. There are

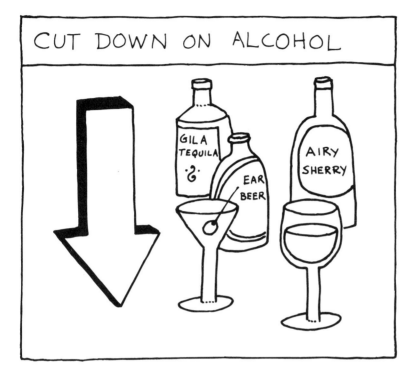

roughly 10 million alcoholics in the United States. Personality differences, family background, and biochemical individuality must explain why some people are addicted to heavy drinking, and why others feel toxic effects after small amounts.

There are several negative aspects of alcohol use in menopause and beyond. Alcohol may act as a trigger for hot flashes. Heavy alcohol use has been associated with osteoporosis and fractures in older women for several reasons. Excess alcohol intake prevents bone cells from building new bone. Alcoholics often eat less calcium-rich food and excrete more calcium in their urine. They exercise less, and have more tendency to fall. Menopause may also be more troublesome because of the toxic effects of alcohol on the ovaries. In general, middle-aged women who have used large amounts of alcohol feel much better when they stop drinking. Nutrition improves when the empty calories of alcohol are replaced by healthy foods high in essential nutrients. Often many other health problems clear up—like excessive fatigue, joint and muscle pains, or hair, skin, and gum problems.

Several recent studies from the United States and Europe have shown an association between alcohol use and breast cancer. Several studies have shown that women drinking 1 or 2 drinks a day are 30-50% more likely to develop beast cancer than nondrinkers. The increased risk is found regardless of whether or not the woman had other risk factors for breast cancer such as a family history of the disease or a late first birth. The link between alcohol and breast cancer may be the finding that alcohol increases estrogen levels in a woman's blood. It is ironic that a substance that decreases risk for heart disease and osteoporosis may increase risks for a dreaded cancer.

Alcohol has been connected to high blood pressure when it is used in regular high doses. Anyone with a blood pressure problem would do well to drink only lightly, if at all.

Alcoholic beverages are made with many chemicals unknown to the consumer, since the federal government has consistently resisted enforcing labeling requirements for the wine, beer, and liquor industries. These chemicals may cause allergy, heart problems, or other illness in susceptible people. This is another reason to use alcohol with caution.

On the whole, it is best to be very careful with drinking in middle age. Analyze your drinking habits, and think about alternatives. Consider exercise, relaxation training, or counseling instead, if you feel you must drink daily to relax, enjoy dinner, or go to sleep. When you do drink, try not to exceed 5 ounces of wine, 12 ounces of beer, or 1 ounce of hard liquor. If alcohol gives you heart palpitations (brandy and red wine can do this), or makes you dizzy or hung over, avoid it! Your body can't recuperate as easily in middle age, and must be treated with respect. Finally, if you do have a compulsion to drink heavily or other problems with alcohol use, don't drink at all. Go to Alcoholics Anonymous instead.

Caffeine

Caffeine is a stimulant found in coffee, black and green tea, chocolate, many soft drinks, and some medicines. It affects the body in numerous ways, and is another recreational drug to be treated with caution. Most adults in our society use caffeine daily and are addicted to some degree to its stimulant properties. If deprived of caffeine, they may suffer mild to severe withdrawal symptoms, including fatigue, headache, irritability, and anxiety. These symptoms last from 1-4 days, and then leave entirely.

Many people enjoy the effects of caffeine, and like the taste of coffee or tea. Is this a safe drug in middle age? What are its pros and cons for the menopausal woman?

Caffeine is used because it decreases fatigue, and stimulates the mind and body to work faster. People think faster and often talk more under its influence. Caffeine enables people to concentrate harder and work longer at many mental and physical tasks.

In high doses, however, caffeine can cause excessive tension and irritability. Meditation and states of relaxation are more difficult under the influence. Users become edgy and uncomfortable, and overreact to stimuli. Their hearts beat faster; they may feel irregular extra beats as thumps in the chest. Blood pressure rises. Sleep is impaired, and a state of fatigue follows. This can make people use more caffeine and perpetuate the problem. All of these drug effects are more pronounced with aging.

Caffeine stimulates the smooth muscle of the gastrointestinal tract, causing some people to have diarrhea. Hence it should not be used at all by people with problems like inflammatory bowel disease (ulcerative colitis or Crohn's disease). Other people with chronic constipation use caffeine as a laxative. The same effect can be obtained, however, with a high-fiber diet of whole grains, beans, vegetables, and added flax seed or bran.

Menopausal women frequently say caffeinated beverages increase hot flashes, and find that eliminating or decreasing caffeine gives them considerable relief from this symptom.

Caffeine has been associated with the development of benign breast lumps in women. It appears to stimulate certain cellular growth factors in the breast, giving rise to more lumpiness and breast pain before periods. When women with breast lumps give up caffeine, the problem often regresses remarkably after 4-6 months. No relationship to breast cancer has been detected.

Caffeine, specifically coffee drinking, has been related to calcium loss in women. It is apparently one factor that can lead to osteoporosis, especially if added to other risk factors. Adding milk to your diet counteracts at least some of this effect (see Chapter 7).

In menopause and in the second half of life, it is good to be tuned in to one's body messages. When you're tired, it is better to rest than to artificially stimulate yourself with a drug. Following the normal ebb and flow of the body's energies leads to a more peaceful and productive life. I suggest limiting coffee to 1 cup a day, or switching to tea, and completely giving up soft drinks (see Chapter 7). Some people find they can easily do without caffeine, and enjoy drinking herbal teas or cereal-based drinks like Postum or Cafix, that resemble coffee but are made from roasted grains. Others drink decaffeinated coffee; best are beans or instant coffee powder from which the caffeine is extracted by a process using hot water rather than chemical solvents.

The news about green and black tea is very promising. Substances in tea known as *polyphenols* have been shown to be powerful inhibitors of cancer in experimental animals—cancers of the skin, lung, esophagus, stomach, small intestine, colon, liver, pancreas and breast have all been prevented or limited in growth by tea. Green tea may be more effective than black, but both look helpful, as does decaffeinated tea. So far the evidence for prevention in humans is only preliminary, but looks very interesting. Tea may also contain substances that protect against heart attack. Do not drink tea that is boiling hot, as this can damage your esophagus (swallowing tube). It looks as though the Asian diet has again been shown to have a great deal of wisdom. When you want a mild and delicious stimulant, tea is clearly the drink of choice.

MAKING CHANGES IN YOUR DIET

A last thought on eating is that everyone makes changes according to his or her own timetable. Most of us do better when changes are gradual, and when we emphasize the positive rather than feel deprived. When I want something sweet and rich, I treat myself to some dates and roasted almonds instead of a candy bar. If I were to miss an old-fashioned hamburger, I would substitute a grilled tofu burger on a whole-wheat bun with lettuce, tomato, sliced onion, mustard, ketchup and a little low-fat mayonnaise! A slow transition to a more plant-based diet is the key, with attention to your individual likes and dislikes. The menus and recipes in the following pages may give you some new ideas, and the bibliography at the end of this book lists helpful references on healthy eating.

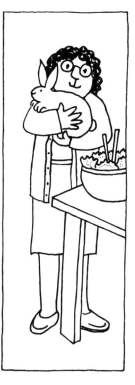

At 45, Lois had two experiences that shook her severely. Her brother had a serious heart attack, and she was operated on for a ruptured appendix. While recuperating in the hospital, Lois asked her doctor why she might have developed appendicitis. "Many people link this problem with a diet low in fiber," her doctor answered. "Appendicitis rarely occurs among people in Africa who eat large amounts of grains and vegetable foods." Lois thought of her own perpetual dieting on cottage cheese, hard-boiled eggs, and meats—with occasional binges on cookies or ice cream. She found out while in the hospital that her serum cholesterol was 250, which worried her because of her brother's heart attack. Her doctor, who was very nutrition-conscious, told her to bring her cholesterol value down below 180 to avoid the family pattern of heart disease. As she lay in bed, Lois realized a whole new way of eating was in order for her. She called a friend at work whom she had considered a health nut, and learned about the benefits of unfamiliar things like sprouted whole-wheat bread, rolled oats, and soybeans. Ultimately she found it easier to lose weight with this diet than it had been with her hard-boiled eggs and meat. A year later her cholesterol level was well below 200, and Lois had become a health nut in her brother's eyes! She was trying to persuade him to try lentil soup and salad instead of steak and french fries. "I draw the line at rabbit food," he would say. "Better to be a healthy rabbit than a man with a second heart attack," was Lois' answer.

High in Calcium

1 c	nonfat milk	300 mg
1 c	1% fat milk	350 mg
1 c	yogurt	300 mg
1 c	calcium-fortified orange juice	320 mg
1 c	calcium-fortified soy milk	300 mg
½ c	low-fat cottage cheese	60 mg
¼ lb	tofu (soybean curd)	150 mg
2	corn tortillas	120 mg
1	medium orange (not juice)	50 mg

Try to eat foods with at least 300 mg of calcium at breakfast

Suggestions for healthy breakfast foods

Whole-grain cereals

Hot: Oatmeal (not the instant kind)
Roman Meal
Wheatena
Zoom

Cold: Shredded wheat
Puffed wheat or rice
Grape Nuts
Uncle Sam
Any other cold cereal made without added sugars or oil (read the label to be sure)

Milk products

Nonfat or 1% fat milk
Nonfat or low-fat yogurt
Low-fat cottage cheese or part-skim ricotta
Soy milk or soy yogurt

Fruit

Oranges, apples, bananas, fresh fruits in season
Raisins and dates to sweeten cereal—instead of sugar
Unsweetened fruit spreads or mashed dates for toast—instead of jam

Whole-grain breads

> Any bread made with 100% whole-grain
> wheat flour or mixed whole-grain flours or
> sprouts
> Whole-grain English muffins
> Whole-grain pancakes or waffles
> Corn tortillas—heat briefly and fill with
> beans, egg, tofu, or cottage cheese

Tofu (bean curd)

> Eat steamed, scrambled, or grilled; with
> onions, curry, soy sauce, or other flavorings

Eggs

> Boiled or poached (restrict yolks to 3 per week)
> Use egg white to make an omelet with
> chopped vegetables

Suggestions for healthy lunch foods
(*indicates recipes which can be found on pp. 195 to 197)

Whole-grain bread sandwiches

> Add fillings such as tomato, onion, cucumber,
> sprouts, a thin slice of cheese, mashed tofu,
> sesame tahini, sardines, or canned salmon

Salad

> Mix vegetables, beans, sprouts, low-fat
> yogurt, or low-fat cottage cheese

Fruit

> Eat whole or cut-up fruits with plain, low-fat
> yogurt or cottage cheese

Soup

> Lentil, split pea, or other bean with vegetables

Breads

> Corn tortillas
> Whole-grain bread
> Whole-grain crackers without added oil or
> butter (e.g., Ry-Krisp, Wasa Crispbread,
> Finn Crisp, Kavli Flatbread, Siljans Knacke)

Any dinner food listed below

High in Calcium

¼ lb	tofu (soybean curd)	150 mg
1 oz	hard cheese	200 mg
1 c	low-fat cottage cheese	120 mg
1 c	nonfat milk	300 mg
1 c	1% fat milk	350 mg
1 c	calcium-fortified soy milk	300 mg
1 c	low-fat yogurt	300 mg
8	medium canned sardines	350 mg
3 oz	canned salmon with bones	170 mg
2	corn tortillas	120 mg

Try to eat foods with at least 300 mg of calcium at lunch

Suggestions for healthy snack foods

Fresh fruit

Popcorn (air popped, without added butter)

Whole-grain crackers, made without added oil or butter (Ry-Krisp, Wasa Crispbread, Finn Crisp, Kavli Flatbread, Siljans Knacke)

Slices of raw vegetables (carrots, green peppers, zucchini, cucumbers, tomatoes, and other vegetables) with tofu or cottage cheese dip

Plain, low-fat yogurt with fresh or dried fruit

Soy nuts (soak dry soybeans overnight, rinse and spread on oiled cookie sheet. Roast at 350° F, stirring occasionally, until well browned. Season lightly with tamari or salt and store in air-tight container.)

Soy milk shake (blend soy milk (calcium-fortified or plain) with a banana, ice and unsweetened cocoa powder or other flavoring as desired)

Suggestions for healthy dinner foods

(*indicates recipes which can be found on pp. 195 to 197)

Whole-wheat spaghetti
with *tomato-eggplant-garlic sauce, and parmesan cheese or toasted cashews

A "comprehensive salad"
Lettuce, bean sprouts, onion, sliced (raw or cooked green, yellow, and red) vegetables, toasted pumpkin

seeds, sunflower seeds or cashews, cottage cheese, sardines or salmon, with a *low-fat salad dressing. Goes well with baked white or sweet potatoes.

*Brown rice and *stir-fried vegetables*
    with tofu, meat, or fish
Soup
    Lentil, split pea or other bean soup
Dessert
    A bowl of cut-up, fresh fruit topped with yogurt, dates, raisins, toasted sunflower seeds or almonds (a good alternative to ice cream or other sweetened desserts)

High in Calcium

¼ lb	tofu (soybean curd)	150 mg
1 oz	hard cheese	200 mg
1 c	low-fat cottage cheese	120 mg
1 c	nonfat milk	300 mg
1 c	1% fat milk	350 mg
1 c	calcium-fortified soy milk	300 mg
1 c	low-fat yogurt	300 mg
8	medium canned sardines	350 mg
3 oz	canned salmon with bones	170 mg
2	corn tortillas	120 mg
1 c	cooked collard greens	360 mg
1 c	bok choy	230 mg
1 c	kale	210 mg
1 c	mustard greens	180 mg
1	stalk broccoli	160 mg

Try to eat foods with at least 300 mg of calcium at dinner

Recipe suggestions

Lentil, Split Pea, or Bean Soup

A crock pot or slow cooker is ideal for cooking bean soup. Start it at night and it is ready in the morning; start it in the morning and it is ready for dinner. Add 2 cups of water for each cup of beans.

    If you cook beans in a regular pot on the stove, add 3-4 cups of water per cup of beans, and make sure the beans are always covered with water. Keep the pot partially covered—if covered tightly, it may boil over. Follow the directions on p. 167 to prepare beans that do not give you intestinal gas.

Lentils and split peas cook in one to 1-½ hours; larger beans take 3-4 hours.

Add seasonings such as garlic, onion, vegetables, and herbs in the last ½ hour of cooking. Add lemon juice after cooking.

You can add significant calcium content to your soups by cooking them with a stock made from bones or egg shells. Boil bones of meat, poultry, or fish; for every quart of water add 1 tablespoon of vinegar. Simmer the stock for 3-4 hours. Remove the bones and refrigerate the stock overnight. Remove the fat that has hardened, and use the stock or freeze it for future use.

Vegetarians can simmer eggshells in water with added vinegar for 1 hour. Wrap them in cheesecloth, or strain broth before using.

Adding vinegar causes calcium to dissolve out of the bones or eggshells and enter the stock. The result is a low-fat calcium broth for people who don't like or cannot use milk products.

Low-Fat Salad Dressings and Dips

Make your own salad dressings with infinite variations in a blender. The basic ingredient is 1 cup of low-fat yogurt, butter-milk, or cottage cheese. Add a few tablespoons of minced onion, a garlic clove, dill weed, herbal seasonings, curry powder, or dry mustard. Add tomato juice for color and flavor. A tablespoon of olive oil adds richness (optional).

People who do not use milk products can get excellent results with tofu. Put ¼ pound of tofu in a blender, and add ¼ cup of tomato juice, 1 tablespoon of mild vinegar, 1 table-spoon of olive oil (optional), a little soy sauce, tamari or miso paste, and seasonings such as garlic, onion, ginger, curry, or dill weed. Tofu tends to be bland; use more flavorings with it than you would with other bases.

Using less liquid will give you a tasty alternative to tradi-tional party dips—and keep your guests wondering what it is!

For fruit salad, you can make a dressing of yogurt or tofu as a base, and add a banana or other fruit, a date for sweetness, and a dash of cinnamon or vanilla. Blend until smooth.

Tomato-Eggplant-Garlic Sauce

Use a heavy iron skillet or nonstick frying pan, sauté garlic slowly (as many cloves as you wish—the more the better!) in a small amount of olive oil (1 tablespoon or less). Add seasonings such as basil, oregano, thyme, etc. Add a chopped eggplant, chopped fresh tomatoes or unsalted tomato sauce or tomato paste, mushrooms, green peas and other vegetables as desired, and enough water or broth to make the sauce simmer easily. Cover and cook until the eggplant is thoroughly soft, about 20-30 minutes.

Serve over whole-wheat pasta or brown rice.

Top with lightly toasted cashews or sunflower seeds (toast at 300° F for a few minutes) or grated parmesan cheese.

This recipe has many possible variations, depending on the ingredients on hand in your kitchen. It is an example of a low-fat vegetable sauce for pasta or rice. You can add crumbled tofu or cooked beans to increase the protein content. You can add chopped lean meat, fish, or poultry if desired, after the garlic and before the vegetables.

Stir-Fried Vegetable Dishes with Tofu, Meat, or Fish

Using a large, heavy iron skillet or a nonstick frying pan, sauté 2 or 3 cloves of garlic (more if desired) in 1 tablespoon olive oil over low heat. Add chopped ginger root (1 teaspoon or more) if desired. Add tofu cut into cubes, or chopped lean meat, poultry, or fish—about ¼ pound per person, and a little water, stock, or wine to allow the food to simmer and to prevent sticking. Stir frequently, keeping heat low.

After a few minutes, add chopped onion, mushrooms, and assorted chopped vegetables, starting with those which require the most cooking. Add a small amount of liquid, stir, and cover the pan for 1-2 minutes between each addition. If bean sprouts are available, add them at the end, as you turn off the heat.

Serve over brown rice, bulgur wheat, kasha (buckwheat groats), or polenta (corn meal).

Vitamins/Minerals: Yes or No?

16

The most important practical problem confronting us in the nutritional field today is that of learning how to determine the specific nutritional needs of individuals. Typical individuals, as we have seen, have some needs for nutrients that are likely to be far from average.

—Dr. Roger Williams

A health-conscious minority of the population takes vitamin and mineral supplements daily, with the view that their individual needs for certain nutrients may be larger than average, or their diets insufficient. Others consider supplements unnecessary, too troublesome, or too expensive. Nutrition experts often decry the inaccurate claims made for supplements, their potential toxicity in high doses, and the false sense of security they may impart to people whose diets are haphazard. With these viewpoints in mind, here's a simple regimen of supplements suitable for women in and after menopause.

CALCIUM

Calcium is a mineral of great importance to the middle-aged woman, especially if she elects not to use estrogen replacement therapy. If a high-calcium diet is eaten throughout life and calcium supplements (500 mg daily) are begun around age 35, as well as during pregnancy and nursing, women will start menopause with thicker, stronger bones. The decline in bone mass that occurs after menopause (see Chapter 7) will be slower and may not reach the stage where fractures occur. At the time of menopause or at age 50 (whichever comes first) women would do well to take 1,000 mg (1 gram) of calcium daily as a supplement, in addition to getting at least 500 mg daily in their food (see Chapter 15). Take the calcium pills with meals and in divided doses to enhance absorption—for example, take a 500-mg pill with breakfast and another at bedtime. Taking calcium at bedtime may be especially beneficial for your bones.

People taking supplementary calcium sometimes worry about developing calcium deposits in their joints or internal organs. This very rare situation occurs when the parathyroid glands, which regulate calcium levels in the body, are overactive, or when excess vitamin D is ingested. It is not a result of taking calcium supplements, which are safe for the vast majority of people. Women with any serious chronic illness or kidney disease should check with their doctors about any supplements.

Kidney stones made of calcium salts occasionally occur, causing pain and medical problems. However, these stones are not the result of increased calcium intake, except in rare cases, for example where large amounts of antacids are being taken for ulcers. They can be the result of a diet too high in protein or salt, and too low in fluids. The excess protein or salt intake causes a greater loss of calcium in the urine, as explained in Chapter 7. During World War II, when meat was very scarce in England and Europe, cases of kidney stone were rarely seen. After the war, when the diet changed to one rich in meat, kidney stones increased in number.

Many kinds of calcium tablets are currently sold in pharmacies, supermarkets, and health food stores. Most containers list the amount of actual calcium in the tablet; for example, they state that this pill contains 500 mg of calcium. Some brands, however, give the weight of calcium and its accompanying compound, such as calcium carbonate, calcium gluconate, or calcium lactate. In general, calcium carbonate is the best buy, as 1,000 mg (1 gram) of calcium carbonate contains 400 mg of calcium, while 1,000 mg of calcium lactate contains only 130 mg of calcium, and 1,000 mg of calcium gluconate contains only 100 mg of calcium. Not all brands of calcium tablets readily dissolve in the stomach; if they do not do so you may not absorb the calcium you are taking. Try dropping one of your tablets in a glass of vinegar, stir occasionally and wait about 45 minutes. If the tablet has not substantially dissolved by then you should switch to another brand. You can also take chewable calcium tablets, so that you know they have dissolved. Recently calcium has also become available in the form of calcium citrate capsules, which are very easily dissolved and absorbed.

Prices for calcium tablets vary widely. You can pay less than $2 or more than $10 per month for a daily gram of calcium. You might consider a reputable mail-order source of supplements such as Bronson Pharmaceuticals (1945 Craig Road, P.O. Box 46903, St. Louis, MO 63146-6903, telephone: 800-235-3200).

VITAMIN D

Vitamin D is also necessary for calcium absorption; it is formed on our skins by sunlight and found in fortified milk products, fish liver oils, and many multivitamin preparations. About 400 IU are needed daily, but much larger doses can be toxic and should be avoided. Women who do not use milk products should be especially careful to eat other calcium-rich foods and take calcium and vitamin D supplements. Recent research reports indicate that vitamin D plays a major role in bone strength; new forms of this vitamin are being used for the prevention and treatment of osteoporosis in many studies. Vitamin D also plays a role in the prevention of cancer. Be sure to take the right amount of vitamin D daily—400 IU—in a multivitamin or as a separate pill. If you get more through fortified milk or sun exposure this should not be a problem, but avoid over 800 IU daily from your diet and pills.

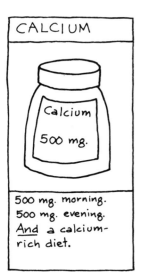

CALCIUM

Calcium

500 mg.

500 mg. morning.
500 mg. evening.
And a calcium-
rich diet.

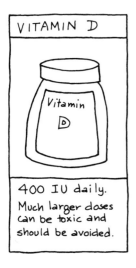

VITAMIN D

Vitamin
D

400 IU daily.
Much larger doses
can be toxic and
should be avoided.

MULTIVITAMINS

Multivitamin and multimineral pills are useful if the amounts of vitamins A and D are not too high (not over 15,000 IU of A or 400 IU of D) and if the doses of minerals are close to the recommended daily allowance. The advantage of taking such a formula is that you are sure of getting most of the essential nutrients you need daily, which your food may or may not supply. Individuals vary in their requirements for essential nutrients, and a vitamin/mineral supplement in addition to a healthy diet may benefit some people whose needs for a particular nutrient are especially high. Considerable work has gone into determining the minimum amount of vitamins and minerals needed to prevent deficiency diseases; nutrition researchers are now also looking at higher amounts that may optimize health, and at the variable needs of different people.

There are several disadvantages to taking a daily multivitamin/mineral supplement which should be considered. They can be expensive, using money which could more effectively be spent for food and other basic needs. Many multivitamin tablets contain iron; if you no longer have monthly bleeding you should not take extra iron—unless your doctor recommends it for anemia or you donate blood. Some people get a false sense of security from supplements, and then subsist on fast food and soft drinks. In so doing, they are overlooking their needs for unrefined carbohydrates and fiber, and missing the amazingly varied protective effects of vegetables and fruits discussed in Chapter 15. They are also ignoring the risks of a diet high in fats and sugars. Finally, some people take huge doses of many vitamins and supplements in a haphazard way, exposing themselves to the risks of toxicity.

I advise postmenopausal women to take a balanced multivitamin pill without iron, containing 400 IU of vitamin D (to help with calcium absorption). Your multivitamin should also contain at least 100% of the RDA for the B vitamins, as vitamins B6, B12 and folic acid have recently been found to protect against high levels of the amino acid homocysteine in the blood. About 12% of the population have inherited a gene that leads to abnormal levels of homocysteine, which can injure

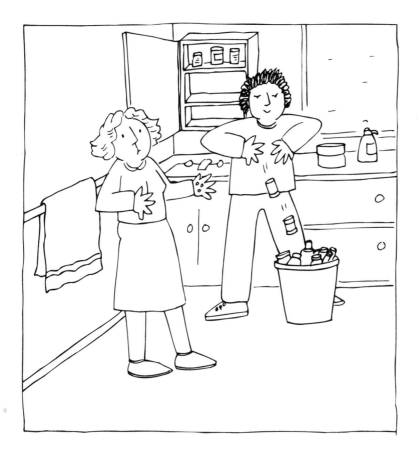

blood vessels and cause heart disease. Folic acid and other B vitamins can give substantial protection. Vegans—vegetarians who do not eat any eggs or milk products—have a special need for vitamin B12.

Many people also benefit from additional "antioxidant" vitamins, which prevent the damage to our cells and genes caused by free radicals formed as our bodies use oxygen. Vitamins A (in the form of beta carotene), C and E perform this role, and may protect against cancer and heart disease. The trace element selenium also functions as an antioxidant, but it should not be used in amounts exceeding 25 to 50 micrograms per day. Many studies have shown the benefits of antioxidant supplements, especially in people with poor nutritional intakes, and a few have failed to show a benefit. In one study of

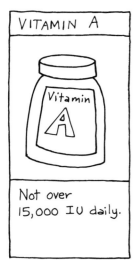

VITAMIN A

Vitamin A

Not over
15,000 IU daily.

male smokers, beta-carotene users fared worse than subjects taking a placebo pill (without any vitamins). More research is underway on this subject. I suggest you read one of the news-letters on nutrition suggested in the last part of this book to keep up to date.

In certain circumstances it is an especially good idea to take vitamin and mineral supplements. People on stringent weight-control programs often do not eat enough to give them-selves the necessary nutrients. People who have lost their appetites because of pain or emotional problems, and patients with chronic diarrhea, alcohol abuse, recent surgery, wounds, burns, or other illness would do well to take daily supple-ments. Consult with your doctor and a nutritionist to help tailor supplements to your particular needs.

Gerrie had a cabinet full of vitamins, minerals, herbal diuretics, and glandular extracts. At one point she took over 20 pills a day for a few months, and then she abandoned them all in disgust. "I'm not sure what I'm doing or if I notice any difference," she said. "The whole thing is confusing and expensive." Gerrie was anxious because she had a mastectomy for breast cancer and wanted to avoid a recurrence. Finally her daughter, who was a nurse, sorted out the cabinet and gave her a simpler regimen. "Mom, you should take 1 multivitamin with vitamin D, your antioxidant pill, and 2 calcium pills with a meal. That's 4 pills a day, and I'm going to throw everything else away." Gerrie groaned as she watched all her expensive pills go in the garbage, but she thought her daughter was right. At least she understood now what to take when and why. She felt more secure taking the 4 pills than she had previously felt taking 20. She decided to eat lots of organically grown vegetables and fruits as her extra insurance.

Catherine lived in a halfway house for alcoholics where the food was inexpensive and rather greasy. White bread, lunch meat, canned veg-etables, and instant mashed potatoes were the rule. She noticed that her hair was falling out easily, her nails broke, and her energy level was low. She rarely took the time to buy any extra food, but she did get a strong multivitamin and mineral pill which seemed to make a lot of difference in how she felt. "This is crazy," she would say to herself each day as she took her pill, "existing on this terrible food and making it up with vitamins. But right now I have no other choice."

Smoking — and Quitting

17

This report points out that the first signs of an epidemic of smoking-related disease among women are now appearing.
—*Dr. Julius B. Richmond, former U.S. Surgeon General*

I am inclined to believe that stopping smoking is very much a personal matter for each one of us. Ultimately, it rests upon a quiet and private decision we make deep within ourselves. Nothing can happen without that decision—not even the most advanced, brilliantly conceived program will work—but everything can happen with it. We each come to that decision in our own way, for our own reasons, and at our own time. There is no time like the present to start saving your own life.
—*Dr. David Geisinger*

Smoking has been mentioned many times in this book. Everyone knows that smoking is connected to cancer of the lung and many other organs, and leads to heart disease and breathing problems in the second half of life. It is less well known that smokers have an earlier menopause, and more problems with brittle bones due to calcium loss (Chapter 7). Smoking is a difficult addiction to overcome, because it is tied in with so many aspects of the smoker's emotional life and daily routines. By midlife, most smokers have used cigarettes

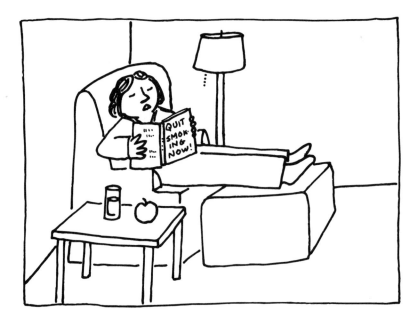

for 20 to 30 years. Yet it is possible to quit—millions of people do so every year. Benefits to your health occur the first day after quitting, and mount over the years. Fifteen years after you quit, your risk of lung cancer is almost as low as someone who has never smoked. And, as far as menopausal symptoms are concerned, ex-smokers report a decrease in severity of hot flashes and a greater sense of well-being.

If you're a smoker, I strongly urge you to begin the task of quitting by becoming aware of each cigarette you smoke, and figuring out why you need it. Are you smoking out of a need for nicotine, out of habit, or because of emotional needs not connected to a real craving for tobacco? Keep records of your findings. When you are ready, begin to think of yourself as a nonsmoker, thereby tuning in to the power of your mind and will to change your life. Get encouragement from nonsmoking friends and loved ones, read a book about quitting, join a group, or take a course with other people who are stopping. Programs to help people quit smoking exist in most areas of the country—some, like Smokers Anonymous, are free. Avail yourself of the counsel and experience of other people if support works for you. Once you have made your resolve, set a date to quit within the next 2 weeks. When the day comes, throw away your cigarettes, ashtrays, and lighters. Stay away from other smokers until you are solid in your convictions. Drink lots of water and juices and practice deep breathing. Take yoga classes, which emphasize deep breathing, stretching, relaxation, and health. Nibble on fruit and raw vegetables rather than candy. Eat healthy food, and don't diet at this time. Don't let your fear of weight gain lure you back into smoking! Tell yourself you will walk them off as your breathing improves, which it will. Regular exercise, such as a walking program, will help diminish cravings for cigarettes and other withdrawal symptoms.

While it's true that most people gain 5 to 10 pounds when they quit smoking, the health benefits of being smoke-free far outweigh the disadvantages of these pounds. Here is some good news about weight—a recent Canadian study showed that most women ex-smokers lose all or most of the extra pounds a few years after quitting. Two years after quitting, the women who quit were less likely to be obese than the smokers.

If you are a heavy smoker and have had severe withdrawal symptoms when trying to quit before, consider asking a doctor to prescribe the nicotine skin patch or nicotine gum. These methods will help you get over the habit of lighting up and will enable your lungs to start healing before you deal with your nicotine addiction. The gum allows you to absorb nicotine through the mucous membranes of your mouth. The patch provides skin absorption of nicotine, and gives a fairly constant nicotine blood level that helps to suppress withdrawal symptoms from cigarettes. The patch or the gum is used for 2-3 months in decreasing doses, until you are able to quit them completely and be free of your nicotine addiction. It is important to quit smoking completely as soon as you begin using the patch or nicotine gum. Most people who have benefited from the gum or the patch have used this method in conjunction with an organized quit-smoking program that gives encouragement, directions and group support. Look for one in your community.

Many people who consider giving up tobacco say something like: "I know I should quit, but I just can't seem to do it."

Take a moment to analyze this statement. Using the word "should" makes it seem that a higher authority is ordering you to do something, and you can frustrate that higher authority by refusing. Using the word "can't" implies that there is an outside power preventing you from changing your behavior. Actually, of course, it's all inside you—the authority, the power, and the will to bring about successful change.

Harriet had been a smoker for over 30 years. She was a brilliant woman, a rapid and creative thinker who had written several books, and who taught a popular history course at the state university. Cigarettes were her constant companion while she read volumes of material, wrote, corrected students' papers, suffered through faculty meetings, and held court at a local coffee house with the campus intellectuals. She punctuated her thoughts with gestures of hand and cigarette. Close as she was to her cigarettes, Harriet knew they were having drastic effects on her health and stamina. Her doctor had loaned her a book on the health consequences of smoking for women, and Harriet understood that her early and difficult menopause might be related to smoking, as well as her shortness of breath and extreme fatigue. Harriet considered herself a hard-core case in terms of her addiction to tobacco, but she also knew that she was a strong and determined person in most other ways. She decided to go to a live-in, stop-smoking program run by the Seventh Day Adventists, in a mountain retreat where there were no cigarettes for sale.

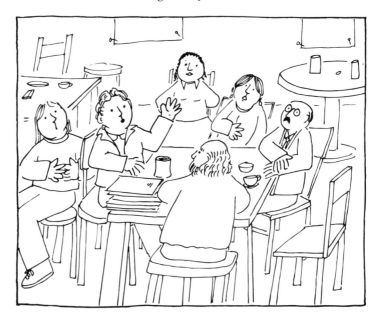

The program was extremely difficult for Harriet, but she appreciated the information, the medical tests, and the group support. She met a 70-year-old man who was attending the program for the third time and intended to succeed this time. By the last day she could walk a mile without stopping or coughing. She set up a buddy system with the older gentleman; they decided to call each other every day to talk about their progress, with S.O.S. calls if they were tempted to smoke. Harriet stayed off cigarettes although it was the hardest thing she had ever done. The next year she organized an elective course on the history of addiction, which was very popular because of her views on the connections between addiction and the profit motive in industrial societies.

Health Care

18

Healing is an equal participation situation—with healer and patient succeeding only if both actively participate in the process.

—Dr. Mike Samuels

For yearly checkups and for illness, it is important to find a medical practitioner with a positive attitude toward women, health, menopause, and self-care measures. You may choose to see a gynecologist, a specialist in internal medicine or a family or general practitioner. Alternatively, you may go to a clinic where you see one of the types of doctors just mentioned or a physician's assistant or nurse practitioner.* It is important that any such health professional be interested in women's medicine, take the time to listen to your problems and questions, and perform a thorough yearly exam including a check of blood pressure, heart and lungs, breasts, abdomen, pelvic

---

*Physician's assistants and nurse practitioners are health professionals trained to assess health and illness, counsel on health practices, and prescribe certain medicines under the supervision of a doctor. They are providing high-quality women's health care in many areas.

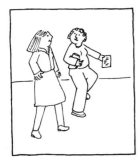

organs, and rectum. Your practitioner should teach you to examine your own breasts. She or he should also be able to advise you on questions concerning drugs, alcohol, smoking, exercise, nutrition and stress. A medical practitioner with an open mind about the benefits and risks of estrogen therapy will enable women to choose what is best for them in this area.

On your part, you should be as clear as possible about your problems, and should keep a written record of when and how much you bleed, as well as any symptoms you may have. You should say that you want information, counseling, physical therapy, or nutritional advice—unless medicine or surgery are absolutely necessary. It is a good idea to write out your questions before an appointment, so you are sure to get them answered. Go to your appointment with a friend who will be your advocate if you are anxious. Feel free to go to another doctor for a second opinion if any treatment is suggested that seems unnecessary to you.

Doctors who take a positive view of menopause, and do not routinely view ill health and pain as inevitable parts of aging, can help women with midlife problems. However, much of medical education has a disease orientation which tends to make doctors pessimistic. Instead of viewing low estrogen levels as nature's norm in the postreproductive years, some doctors say that a woman's vaginal tissues are "estrogen starved," or showing signs of "senile vaginitis." Such attitudes on the part of the doctor can be much more painful than the vaginal problem itself. Hence, it is important for women to find doctors with positive views of the aging process, which is why the newly forming network of menopause clinics in women's health centers is so valuable.

If you do not have any health insurance, find the best free or low-cost clinic in your area. Many Planned Parenthood clinics now treat midlife and menopausal women, or will advise you where to go. Eat a plant-based diet and walk every day, as described in this book, to stay healthy. Vote and lobby for whatever health-care reform plan meets your approval. The plight of uninsured and underinsured people in this country is a serious national problem that will only be solved by vigorous citizen participation.

Choose carefully when you want a counselor for emotional and psychological help. Midlife women should look for a well-trained person (such as a social worker, licensed counselor, psychologist, or psychiatrist) with whom it is comfortable to talk. Look for someone who encourages personal growth as well as helping with emotional pain. This kind of counseling is more helpful for many people than the kind which routinely

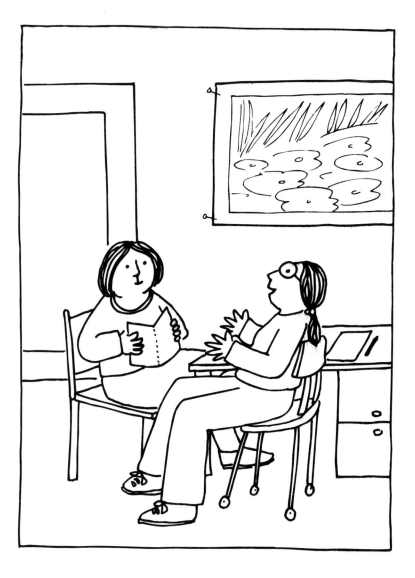

uses tranquilizers or antidepressants. Group therapy and midlife self-help groups are also available in many areas—women in a self-help group in my area call themselves "the red-hot mamas"!

Bernice went to Dr. Williams because of soreness with intercourse. She was nervous about the visit because she had not seen him in 2 years, and she feared he would pressure her to take postmenopausal estrogens as he did with most of his patients. She preferred not to take hormone pills, as her sister had developed breast cancer. Bernice was also anxious because she had met a new man this year, 5 years after her divorce, and she wasn't sure how Dr. Williams would react to her having an affair. She got undressed and, lying on the examining table, waited for him to arrive. When he did a pelvic exam, Dr. Williams remarked that she had a bad case of "vaginal atrophy" and he pointed out the characteristics of the problem to a medical student who was working with him. Bernice felt angry and embarrassed by this episode. She accepted Dr. William's prescription for estrogen tablets in order to get out of his office as quickly as possible. Once home, she cried, punched her pillow, and decided she had to find another doctor.

She found out that a women's center in a nearby city had opened a special service for midlife women. Bernice went there the next week and had quite a different experience. She was given some interesting pamphlets on menopause, sex, aging, and the pros and cons of estrogen therapy. In a relaxed discussion with a nurse practitioner, she found out that she could use a small amount of estrogen cream twice a week and not take pills for her problem of soreness. Above all, she found out that the physical examination did not have to be painful or embarrassing, but could be informative and reassuring. She came away feeling more self-confident and hopeful about her new love affair.

Summing It All Up!

19

I have described numerous paths to the goal of postmenopausal zest, and proposed a positive view of ourselves in midlife. Staying connected to the world; relaxation, exercise, nutrition, supplements; not smoking; and finding good health care—each is an important part of every day we live.

In and after the menopausal years, women have certain special needs, problems, and advantages. Their special needs are for more calcium, more exercise, and more attention to healthful, balanced living. Their special problems are those of hot flashes, vaginal soreness with intercourse, and bone loss. Their special advantages are that the period of life after menopause is smoother—no more premenstrual tension, hormonal mood swings, pelvic aching, or menstrual problems. No more concerns about birth control. Daily life seems to many women to have more balance and steadiness. Postmenopausal zest can become a reality!

In China, the 60th birthday is considered a momentous event, a time when the family gathers to celebrate the status and wisdom of the elder. Other societies which revere age have special positions for older women which acknowledge their worth and power. Aging is seen as a gain in wisdom and not just a loss of youth. Interestingly enough, in these societies,

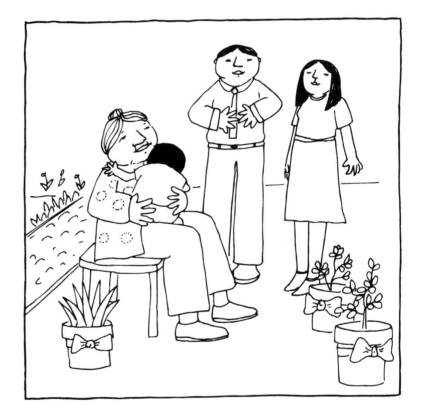

menopause is not viewed as a negative event, but as a time when women rise in social status and enjoy more privileges.

Can this be so in our society? Yes, if we make it so. Although our culture has glorified youth, especially in women, this emphasis is changing. As birthrates stay low and the life span increases, we find an increasing proportion of our citizens in middle- and old-age groups. This phenomenon has been called the "graying of America." Midlife and older people are becoming a stronger social and political force. Two other factors are also at work—the philosophy of personhood and the women's movement.

The philosophy of personhood is an emerging view in our culture; it holds that each person is not only equal but unique, and should develop her or his potential, regardless of age, sex, or ethnic group. We can go back to school in our 50s, take up new interests in our 60s, and change our names or our sexual orientations. This view of life allows midlife women to free themselves from old stereotypes and gain a sense of self-worth. The women's movement does the same thing, and encourages women to use their conviction of equality and power in the world around them—at work, at home, and in their communities and nations. Once women achieve feelings of real self-worth, regardless of age or appearance, they will see middle age or menopause not as a tragedy, but as a time of accumulated wisdom and experience. They can see the second half of life building on the first half and developing from it in new ways.

I have discussed the special needs and problems of midlife in some detail. But what you do with postmenopausal years is the next chapter, for you to write for yourself. Some women need to concentrate on survival or sanity in this difficult world. Others want to develop themselves in new ways they have not yet explored. Your creativity in the arts, writing, business or politics may surprise you if you give it a chance. Some women will become strong figures in their families; others will be more active in their communities once family responsibilities decrease. Some will use their creativity for the good of the planet, which desperately needs more female energy to heal its rifts.

All of us can use role models at this time in life. Notice how many of the Nobel Prizes for peace have recently gone to women: Alva Myrdal of Sweden for her work on disarmament, Mother Teresa of Calcutta for her work with the poor, Mairead Corrigan and Betty Williams of Northern Ireland for their work to stop the fighting in their country, and Daw Aung San Suu Kyi for her work to bring social democracy to Burma. Think about Maya Angelou, the African-American writer and poet who spoke so eloquently at the Clinton inaugural, or Diane Feinstein and Barbara Boxer, U.S. senators from California. All these women have used the special wisdom and experience of being female to inspire their action in the world.

Meredith spoke of her midlife changes very emphatically. "I began to know myself in a new way after the children left home and I turned 50. I saw that my life was limited and yet unlimited at the same time. Limited in that I wouldn't live forever. Unlimited in that I could really be myself for the first time in many years. I decided to put my energies into the political work that had always interested me, and within 2 years I was running for city councilwoman. I feel I can take all my talents in working with and for people, and use them in a larger way in politics. I'd like to see a lot more women, especially older women, getting into community leadership. They've got a lot of wisdom to share."

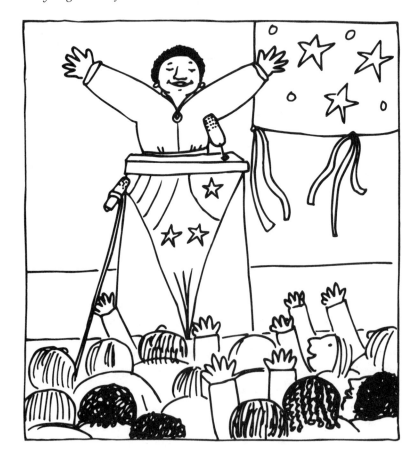

Suggestions for Further Reading

ADOPTION

Martin, C. *Beating the Adoption Game.* Harcourt Brace & Co., 1988. A complete book about adoption, including a section on accelerating the process through private adoptions. Very good on the practical and psychological aspects of adoption.

CANCER

Lerner, M. *Choices in Healing—Integrating the best of conventional and complementary approaches to cancer.* MIT Press, 1994. A unique resource, carefully researched, on finding responsible mind-body, nutritional and alternative approaches which complement standard medical therapy for cancer. Also helpful in choosing and evaluating standard medical treatment in the U.S., Japan and Europe. Written by a MacArthur Prize fellow who founded the Commonweal Cancer Help Program.

Love, S. *Dr. Susan Love's Breast Book.* Addison Wesley Publishing Co., 1995. A comprehensive book on breast cancer and its treatment written by a compassionate surgeon.

EXERCISE

Anderson, B., Burke, E., and Pearl, B. *Getting in Shape.* Shelter Publications, P.O. Box 279, Bolinas, CA 94924, 1994. Graduated programs for stretching, muscle-building and aerobic exercise (including walking) for women and men, written by masters in their field. Excellent pictures, practical advice. Highly recommended.

Cooper, K. H. *The Aerobics Way.* M. Evans & Co., New York, 1977. An explanation of the benefits of vigorous exercise, followed by detailed plans for gradual conditioning for all age groups in a variety of activities (walking, jogging, cycling, swimming, racquet sports, stationary bicycling, stair climbing, rope skipping). Includes plans for the very obese and for people who have had coronary bypass surgery.

Hittleman, R. *Richard Hittleman's Yoga: 28-Day Exercise Plan.* Bantam Books, New York, 1969. A systematic beginner's guide to yoga postures with illustrations of each exercise. Gently leads into flexibility and more peace of mind.

Myers, Leora. *Menopause and Beyond: A Fitness Plan for Life.* Adelaide Press, San Francisco, 1995. An excellent guide to all aspects of fitness: stretching, weight training, aerobics, and more—by an RN fitness instructor with a strong interest in menopause.

GETTING TO KNOW YOURSELF AND EXPLORING YOUR CREATIVITY

Capacchione, L. *The Creative Journal: The Art of Finding Yourself.* Newcastle Publishing Co., 1989. A book on self-discovery through keeping a journal of drawings. Easy and wise.

Goldberg, N. *Writing Down the Bones.* Shambala, 1986. A wonderful short and easy book that frees you to express and understand yourself through writing.

Rogers, N. *The Creative Connection: Expressive Arts as Healing.* Science and Behavior Books, 1993. A book about self-discovery through exploring the connections between movement, art, music and writing—all in the framework of a gentle, person-centered approach.

MENOPAUSE

Beyene, Y. *From Menarche to Menopause: Reproductive Lives of Peasant Women in Two Cultures.* State University of New York Press, 1989. A woman anthropologist describes the different experience of menopause among Mayans in southern Mexico and rural Greek islanders—a fascinating cross-cultural analysis.

Cobb, J. O. *Understanding Menopause.* Penguin/Plume, 1993. A thorough and reassuring Canadian book on menopause. Janine Cobb, the author, also publishes *A Friend Indeed*, an excellent newsletter on menopause (see Newsletters at the end of this bibliography).

Cutler, W. B., et al. *Menopause, A Guide for Women and the Men Who Love Them.* W.W. Norton & Company, New York, 1992. A scholarly book on menopausal problems favoring hormone use, and providing a thorough discussion of its benefits and risks.

Lock, M. *Encounters with Aging: Mythologies of Menopause in Japan and North America.* University of California Press, 1993. A woman anthropologist reports on her 20-year study of menopause in Japan and North America; highly recommended.

Taylor, D. and Sumrall, A. (eds). *Women of the 14th Moon.* The Crossing Press, Freedom, CA, 1991. A collection of 90 short poems and personal stories on menopause from wonderfully diverse perspectives—entertaining, illuminating and comforting.

Voda, A. M., Dinnerstein, M., O'Donnell, S.R. (eds). *Changing Perspective on Menopause.* University of Texas Press, Austin, 1982. A collection of essays by contemporary scholars on menopause, from an anthropologic, literary, psychological, and physiological perspective. Excellent original material.

Voda, A. M., *Menopause, Me and You.* Booklet available by writing to Dr. Ann Voda, College of Nursing, 25 South Medical Drive, Salt Lake City, UT 84112. Excellent information on hot flashes and other aspects of menopause, not oriented to hormone use.

NEWSLETTERS ON HEALTH TOPICS AND AGING

A Friend Indeed. P.O. Box 1710, Champlain, NY 12919-1710. A lively, informative, sharing newsletter, exploring menopause as mythology, biology, and feelings.

Harvard Women's Health Watch. P.O. Box 420234, Palm Court, FL 32142-0234. A very informative newsletter from Harvard Medical School, covering many aspects of women's health; generally has an open-minded attitude towards alternative and complementary medicine.

Hot Flash: Newsletter for Midlife and Older Women. P.O. Box 816, Stony Brook, NY 11790-0609. A newsletter devoted to promoting postmenopausal zest by giving information on the health, mental needs, and resources of older women. Women's health column is written by Dr. Sadja Greenwood, the author of this book.

Menopause News. 2074 Union St., San Francisco, CA 94123. A popular national newsletter on all aspects of menopause, including book reviews and letters from readers.

Nutrition Action Healthletter. Center for Science in the Public Interest (CSPI), Suite 300, 1875 Connecticut Ave., N.W., Washington DC 20009-5728. A monthly magazine on practical nutritional information and the political battles for consumer education about food and health. Witty, well illustrated, and easy to read.

The Soy Connection—Health and Nutrition News about Soy, 10525 N.W. Ambassador Dr., Suite 202, Kansas City, MO 64153. For those interested in new research on soy foods, and how they may promote health.

University of California, Berkeley Wellness Letter. P.O. Box 420148, Palm Coast, FL 32142. A lively, monthly newsletter giving the latest on nutrition, fitness and stress management—for men, women and families.

NUTRITION

Brody, J. *Jane Brody's Good Food Book.* Bantam Books, New York, 1987. A wonderful source book on nutrition and healthy foods, with recipes low in fat and salt, written by a *New York Times* science writer.

McDougall, M. *The McDougall Health Supporting Cookbooks: Volumes One & Two.* New Win Publishing, Inc., 1985. Vegan (no meat, eggs or dairy) recipes designed for health and convenience in cooking. The author's husband is a doctor who has written widely on prevention and health.

Messina, M. and V. *The Simple Soybean and Your Health.* Avery Publishing Group, 1994. A fascinating and accessible book explaining new findings in soy research, relevant to breast cancer, heart disease, osteoporosis, and other problems. Includes recipes and ways to use soy foods.

Shulman, M.R. *Fast Vegetarian Feasts: The Revised Edition with Fish.* Doubleday and Co., New York, 1986. Healthy and delicious recipes, low in fat and salt, prepared in 45 minutes or less.

Wasserman, D. *Simply Vegan: Quick Vegetarian Meals.* Available through the Vegetarian Resource Group, P.O. Box 1463, Baltimore, MD 21203. A short, easy cookbook that gives nutritional information and the calcium content of all recipes.

SEXUALITY

Barbach, L. *Sex after Fifty,* available by calling 415-383-0755. An enjoyable videotape made by women psychologists and doctors, discussing how women and men can keep a sexual relationship going for a lifetime.

Barbach, L., et al. *Shared Intimacies: Women's Sexual Experiences.* Anchor Press/Doubleday, Garden City, NY, 1980. An excellent book of interviews with women of all ages about their sexual experiences. The author, a psychologist and sex therapist, includes interesting, diverse material on sex in menopause and beyond.

Blank, J. *Good Vibrations: Mail Order Catalog,* 1210 Valencia St., San Francisco, CA 94110. A woman-owned business devoted to sexual pleasure and information. The catalog lists vibrators, sex toys, condoms, and many good books and videos relating to women's sexual problems and pleasures. Highly recommended.

SMOKING

Ferguson, T. *The Smoker's Book of Health.* G. P. Putnam's Sons, New York, 1987. A very practical guide for smokers on how to lower your risks even while smoking, and how to quit when you're ready, written by a physician.

Gahagan, D. *Switch Down and Quit.* Ten Speed Press, Berkeley, CA, 1987. A very savvy book on nicotine addiction and how to overcome it, and on the role of cigarette advertising in maintaining your addiction.

Wanning, E. *Meditations for Surviving Without Cigarettes.* Avon Books, 1994. A day-by-day book to help quitters through 365 days without smoking. Contains tips for outwitting the urge, a wide range of medical facts, assurances of a brighter life that lies ahead, and inspirational quotes from literary and celebrity figures.

STRESS AND RELAXATION

Benson, H. *The Relaxation Response.* Avon, New York, 1975. An excellent short book by a Harvard physician on how and why to make a daily habit of relaxation.

Ornish, D. *Dr. Dean Ornish's Program for Reversing Heart Disease.* Ballantine Books, New York, 1990. A pioneering book on nutrition, exercise and stress reduction to prevent or treat heart disease, by one of the first doctors to study and demonstrate that such a program is effective. The relaxation exercises are widely applicable, and the recipes are excellent.

Rossman, M. *Healing Yourself: A Step-by-step Program for Better Health Through Imagery.* Walker and Co., 1987. A wise and accessible book on how to use imagery for relaxation and access to your own solutions for problems.

URINARY PROBLEMS AND INCONTINENCE

Burgio, K., et al. *Staying Dry: A Practical Guide to Bladder Control.* The Johns Hopkins University Press, Baltimore and London, 1989. A best-selling paperback book that explains incontinence and gives an action plan that helps 90% of the people who try it, based on muscle strengthening and the timing of urination.

Chalker, R., et al. *Overcoming Bladder Disorders.* Harper & Row, 1990. An excellent book, co-authored by a woman urologist, explaining incontinence and many other urinary tract problems in women and men, and giving medical and self-help solutions.

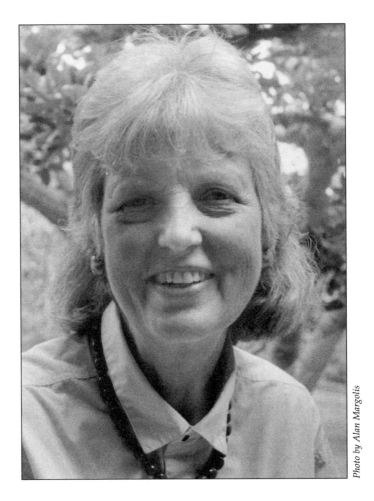

Photo by Alan Margolis

Sadja Greenwood, M.D., M.P.H., describes herself as a "62-year-old woman doctor, mother of two grown sons, and a slow jogger, looking for the truths about life and the joy in every day." Dr. Greenwood gives lectures and conducts seminars on menopause and midlife zest. In her teaching and practice, she strives to combine advances in scientific medicine with natural methods of self-healing such as walking, stretching, swimming and a healthy, plant-based diet. She is an Assistant Clinical Professor at the University of California Medical Center in San Francisco.

Order Form

____ **The Counselor's Guide to Learning to Live Without Violence** $29.95
by Daniel Jay Sonkin, Ph.D., hardcover

____ **Family Violence and Religion:** An Interfaith Resource Guide $29.95
Compiled by the Volcano Press staff, hardcover

____ **The Physician's Guide to Domestic Violence:** *How to ask* $10.95
the right questions and recognize abuse . . . another way to save a life
by Patricia R. Salber, M.D. and Ellen Taliaferro, M.D.

____ **Learning to Live Without Violence:** *A Handbook for Men* $14.95
by Daniel Jay Sonkin, Ph.D. and Michael Durphy, M.D.

____ **Learning to Live Without Violence:** *A Worktape for Men* $15.95
(2 C-60 cassettes)

____ **Sourcebook for Working with Battered Women** $17.95
by Nancy Kilgore

____ **Every Eighteen Seconds:** *A Journey Through Domestic Violence* $8.95
by Nancy Kilgore

____ **Battered Wives** by Del Martin $12.95

____ **Conspiracy of Silence:** *The Trauma of Incest* $12.95
by Sandra Butler

____ **Menopause, Naturally:** *Preparing for the Second Half of Life* $14.95
Updated, by Sadja Greenwood, M.D., M.P.H.

____ **Menopausia Sin Ansiedad.** Spanish edition of $14.95
Menopause, Naturally

____ **Period.** With removable parent's guide $9.95
by JoAnn Gardner-Loulan, Bonnie Lopez and Marcia Quackenbush

____ **La Menstruacion.** Spanish edition of *Period.* $9.95

____ **Lesbian/Woman** by Del Martin and Phyllis Lyon, hardcover $25.00

(continued on next page)

To order directly, please send check or money order for the price of the book(s) plus $4.50 shipping charge for the first book, and $1.00 for each additional book ordered to Volcano Press, P.O. Box 270-05, Volcano, CA 95689-0270, or you may order by phone with a VISA or MasterCard by calling toll-free 1-800-879-9636.

California residents please add 7.25% sales tax.

Volcano Press books are available at discounts for bulk purchases, professional counseling, educational, fund-raising or premium use. Free catalogs are available. Please call or write for details.

Please send Volcano Press catalogs to:

Name: _____

Address: _____

City, State, Zip: _____